YOGA AND COMMON SENSE

YOGA AND COMMON SENSE

Revised Edition

INA MARX

THE BOBBS-MERRILL COMPANY, INC.
INDIANAPOLIS   NEW YORK

Designed by Dan Kirklin
Manufactured in the United States of America

First printing

Library of Congress Cataloging in Publication Data

Marx, Ina.
  Yoga and common sense.

  Includes index.
  1. Yoga.   I. Title.
B132.Y6M34 1977   613.7   79-98294
ISBN 0-672-52269-1

I dedicate this book to all my students

CONTENTS

ILLUSTRATIONS OF EXERCISES

Photographs by Diana Bryant

PREFACE

*"Life begins at forty"—we read it, we write it, we talk about it,
but most of us don't believe a word of it. I can vouch for the
truth of that statement, because I first began Yoga when I was
forty. Now, at forty-plus, I am living and enjoying life as I
never have, as we were created to: with good health, peace of
mind and happiness.*

These were the opening words of the first edition of *Yoga
and Common Sense*, contradicting the generally accepted
idea of the American public that forty is the downhill age. We
were then at the peak of the youth rebellion; it was the era of
the rock music explosion, of pop and pot culture, of the
miniskirt and the topless torso. The battle cry was "Don't trust
anyone over thirty," and the self-confidence of the aging
citizen had reached its bottom mark.

At forty-plus I was experiencing a rebirth through Yoga. I
thrilled at my new-found good health and good figure, increased energy and stamina, and the discovery that life can
really be beautiful and that age has absolutely nothing to do
with it.

"You are as old as you feel" and "You are as young as you
look" were clichés that took on new meaning. Coué's famous
confidence-enforcement slogan, "Every day in every way I am
getting better and better," became a reality. I had gotten a new
lease on life through Yoga, and I intended to hold on to it; and
it did take effort in the beginning. I had to readjust my home

life in order to incorporate Yoga into my daily life, and it wasn't easy. My youngest daughter was still living at home and needed a lot of chauffeuring about; and my husband, although resigned more or less, thought of Yoga as a rival in our marriage. In practice I sometimes pushed too hard, pulling or straining muscles, and became impatient. It took time for me to acknowledge my structural limitations and the inherent weaknesses of my back—not to accept them as limitations, but to learn to work around them.

As the demands of my Yoga teaching grew from day to day, I had to come to terms with myself on just how much I wanted to become involved. I had started teaching Yoga in my basement with a contingent of six reluctant neighbors, and then, as my confidence increased, I applied at various Ys to teach. Eventually I started out on my own, rented my first little studio, progressed to a bigger one, and finally made my life's dream a reality by establishing a complete Yoga center.

There came a time when I got swept up into the pseudospiritual wave of Yoga as it is written about in most Yoga books and practiced by most Yoga societies in the United States: the hang-up on ritual, long meditation, chanting, recitation on prayer beads, and involvement in deep Yoga philosophy. I envied those who could devote their whole lives to Yoga, and I experienced pangs of guilt for my material existence, which is contrary to all the Yoga teachings that impose abstinence and detachment from mundane needs and desires.

I had to come to grips with myself and face the facts that I am neither an ascetic nor a Spartan, that I truly enjoy the material comforts that life has to offer, and that I need not experience any feelings of guilt. I try to impress on my students today that we are not Indians or Hindus, that we were born into a Western twentieth-century material civilization, and that we cannot devote our lives to Yoga rituals and meditation. But we can adapt Yoga and incorporate it into a small

portion of our daily lives to enrich them and to help us cope
with them, not to "turn off" but to "tune in." In my realm of
teaching, I have tried and have succeeded in taking the "Eastern mystique" out of Yoga, stripping it of its esoteric and
mystical implications, and presenting it as neither a religion
nor a cult, but as a superb and unfailing scientific method to
achieve total well-being for body and mind.

I am now fifty-plus at this writing, and Yogas has indeed
fulfilled the things I thought it would. I accept that there is a
chronological aging process, but I do not accede to it. Except
for a few wrinkles around the eyes, I truly believe that I am
getting younger. I feel younger today than I did at twenty-five.
I feel stronger, more energetic, more vital and more optimistic. I look forward to each day as a new discovery. I have come
to savor each pleasure that life has to offer, and I have discovered a new world of pleasure through Yoga. I have truly
learned (and it was difficult indeed) to live in the present, to
accept the past as a memory, and to view idle speculation
about the future as unproductive. Yoga teaches you that only
the present is true reality, and it is only when you truly live in
the present that life becomes enjoyable.

I look good, and although there are certain inheritance
factors (I am blessed with good skin and I have no gray hair), I
attribute my generally youthful appearance to Yoga. Both my
figure and my muscle tone belie my age, and, generally speaking, I present the best advertisement for Yoga. People are
usually surprised when they learn my age, and those who
haven't seen me for a long time invariably remark that I look
better than I looked when they last saw me.

I feel great and hardly ever get sick. Even though I have
physical problems which others might succumb to, I function
well at all times. I have learned through Yoga to become
attuned to my body and to listen to it, and though I generally
practice Yoga daily, I leave it up to my body whether to

practice an hour (which is my usual routine) or exceed an hour, or to practice ten minutes or not at all. I need very little sleep today, I really never feel tired, and I have boundless energy and stamina.

My school, Yoga for Long Island, teaches 300 to 350 students per week. I have several teachers working for me, but I teach all the advanced classes myself and give monthly meditation instruction and special breathing classes. I have recently opened Yoga for Manhattan and commute twice a week to give classes there. I train all my teachers personally, and since I am a perfectionist in Yoga, this requires great effort and diligence.

At our center we hold seminars with visiting Yoga teachers from all over the world in order to keep up with all the latest Yoga techniques, and I am constantly working on improving my teaching. I take courses whenever I can on related subjects such as anatomy, kinesiology, body massage, psychology and hypnotism. I attend Yoga workshops in various cities in the United States, and once a year I fly to France to work with the special teacher from whom I take lessons.

We do volunteer work teaching Yoga to mental patients, drug addicts, the physically disabled, and alcoholics. I guest-lecture to organizations, at colleges and high schools. I was among the first to introduce Yoga to high school children, and I am happy to hear that it is now integrated into many schools.

Although only my husband and I are at home now, I still have household duties to perform and shopping to do, and I do all my own cooking. There is entertaining for my husband's business friends, there are mutual interests to be pursued, and we travel together whenever we have a chance. I seem to have time for everything I want to accomplish, and an unlimited supply of energy to carry it through.

Yoga has helped me overcome serious hurdles during the

past few years. I shudder to think what my life would have
been like without Yoga.

To me, life represents progress and achievement. I feel that
only in these things lie fulfillment and happiness. The keys
are self-confidence and self-acceptance. Self-confidence is
the root of all our striving. We may think we desire material
riches, personal gain, or the approval of others to make us
happy, but even when we attain them, we are neither content
nor happy. Only within ourselves can we find happiness. I
gained self-confidence by accomplishing what I thought was
impossible. For various people there are different areas of
accomplishment, depending on their inclinations. For some
it is in the arts, painting or music or writing; for others it is in
education or handiwork or even baking a perfect cake. For me
it lies in physical endeavor. The fact that I am able to perform
and hold intricate Yoga positions never fails to thrill me and
to inspire me to try harder. It took me ten years, for instance, to
accomplish the Scorpion position, and it is a source of un-
equaled pride for me.

Yoga imposes self-discipline and presents challenge, and
those are the keys to youth and longevity. As long as you keep
working and striving you can never grow old either physically or mentally. Your body and mind cannot deteriorate if
you keep them at the peak of condition. The ravages of old age
can take hold only in stagnation. The idea of Yoga is to
increase activity, instead of decreasing it to accommodate the
aging process.

I don't intend to get old. I am looking forward to writing
about Yoga at sixty-plus and seventy-plus, and I intend to
stand on my head at eighty and have a ball.

YOGA AND COMMON SENSE

1

WHY
YOGA?

Why Yoga in preference to other physical exercise?

Why Yoga instead of other mental-improvement programs?

I will do my very best to prove to you that the practice of Yoga is unique, superior and totally encompassing; that it is a physical, mental and spiritual experience all in one; and that when you accept it, you don't need to look further. Fitness today is very much "in" in the United States. It is heralded, advocated and preached by educators, physicians, and even presidents, and it is advertised, packaged, and sold by profiteers. Each one has his particular idea or brand of fitness, and those most successful in pushing their brainchild or product have either social or political influence or the financial capacity to spend large sums on advertising.

There exists not one overall idea as to what technique leads to or constitutes fitness. The general public will bounce from one exercise program to the next, and thus we have gone in recent years from isometrics to isokinetics, from aerobics to Air Force exercises, from jogging to t'ai chi chuan. Included in this crusade for fitness, and an unfortunate testimony to the poor physical shape of Americans as a whole, are walking, hiking, swimming, bicycling, tennis and golf, which in other westernized countries are considered natural activities of everyday life. Some educators advise daily walks as an adequate fitness program, and for many sedentary citizens who move only from the office to the car to the home and exchange one sitting or lying position for another, walking for the sake of walking becomes a source of revelation.

Americans are also "instant" geared: instant food, instant medicine, instant bliss. We will try almost anything that requires a minimum of effort. Any diet, course, book, record or tape that promises results in a short time has a good chance of being a best seller as, for example, the current book with ample scientific evidence that to keep yourself physically fit you need spend only thirty minutes a week on exercise. However, this is the barest minimum to keep the skeletal and muscular systems from disintegration.

Most large cities offer a wealth of physical-fitness programs. Every conceivable type of exercise—rhythm, dance, stretch, body movement—is available. There are gyms galore featuring every conceivable gadget and machine to mold and contour you and lead you to everlasting health and beauty. Each program, of course, claims to be superior to all other existing methods. There are differences in name and application, but they have these drawbacks in common: (a) with very few exceptions, it is not feasible to do them alone; (b) you can perform them only at their particular location, and (c) they are all expensive. Health Clubs and Y's offer free exercise classes, but the yearly membership is usually quite steep.

I enjoy all physical activity, and I have an insatiable curiosity. I'm as easily swayed as the next person by advertisements, and as easily convinced by someone who swears by a particular fitness method. I have exercised, dancercised and sexercised to rock music, drums and gongs. I have stretched, bounced, shaken and wiggled. I have even tumbled (which was quite careless of me, to say the least, and I suffered deeply for it by throwing my uncertain back out of condition). I have swung from trapezes, hung on bars, slanted on slantboards. I have let myself be buckled and strapped into the most unbelievably weird machines and have allowed myself to be stretched and pulled and manipulated.

I cannot, of course, list individually all the exercise programs available, but to sum up: some were fun, most were boring; some were valid, most were not.

I am sure that any program pursued on a regular basis will bring results in fitness, weight loss, well-being, etc., but none of them can be easily pursued at home and incorporated into one's life. When the course has ended, sooner or later the enthusiasm wanes and all accomplishments evaporate.

Of great popularity today are the martial arts imported from the East—judo, jiujitsu, karate, aikido, kung fu and t'ai chi chuan. Their movements range from slow to fast and are used as self-defense and feats of strength, and generally promote great physical fitness. Many of them, however, require a preexisting degree of good physical condition and are mostly applicable to very young people. Because of this current vogue, many unorthodox Occidentals who are unfit to teach are hanging out shingles, and I have heard of many instances in which people have been badly hurt.

I very much advise judo or jiujitsu or karate as an excellent fitness program for young people, because each of them will promote physical agility, strength and endurance and will inspire confidence and harmony of mind. However, one should exercise discrimination in choosing a teacher. A conscientious teacher will always start the lesson with warm-up exercises—accelerated Yoga movements, for example—to prevent injuries to the body. Martial arts, as well as some other practices from the East, such as acupuncture and shiatsu, which are seen in the West as monumental breakthroughs in obtaining health and fighting disease, are innate to Oriental culture and part of everyday life. T'ai chi chuan, for instance, which is taught privately or in schools as an intricate body movement, is very much part of the Eastern scene. All over China you can see people, especially old men, performing the movements like shadow-boxing, and no one pays any attention to them. I studied t'ai chi chuan and found it to be lovely and graceful and very relaxing, and excellent for spinal health and posture, but it is extremely difficult to learn. I practiced faithfully every day for two years, then stopped for three months for lack of time, and when I tried to resume it, my body and mind went completely blank. If I should ever resume it, I would have to start again from the very beginning.

I have also been Mensendiecked, Alexandered, Feldenkraised and Rolfed. All four systems are very much in vogue today. They are related in the sense that they stress proper posture and body alignment. All those I have met who are teaching these methods are extremely devoted, swear to the infallibility of these disciplines, proclaim them to be the cure for every physical and mental problem or deficiency, and strongly denounce any other type of fitness program.

Mensendieck was invented by Dr. Beth Mensendieck in the early 1900s. She was an American doctor specializing in musculatory imbalances, and her exercises were designed to promote perfect posture in sitting, standing and walking, and to cure and prevent many back diseases. They are done in front of a three-way mirror, preferably in the nude. I have no doubt that they are beneficial if correctly done and consistently practiced. (I practiced faithfully for a while, until boredom took over.) The exercises are extremely concise and very tedious, but they have found great acclaim in Europe, especially in Germany.

The *Alexander* technique is very closely related to Mensendieck and was developed by F. M. Alexander, an Australian, also early in the 1900s. This technique also claims to alleviate back problems, eliminate physical and mental tensions, and, through "Primary Control," achieve a specific relationship of head and neck that leads to perfect posture and carriage. It is not exercise per se. The course consists of corrective manipulation and verbal instructions and is supposed to be practiced as an everyday movement. I finished the course and made an attempt to practice but found it a crashing bore. Since it has been around for such a long time and has so many testimonials praising it, the technique likely does work for its devotees.

The *Feldenkrais* exercises, or functional integration, are the brainchild of Israeli-born Moshe Feldenkrais. I tried them in Israel years ago. They are part of the Esalen culture, and I understand they are now being taught in New York. They are performed lying on the floor, generally on the side, with an instructor directing every move and asking you to isolate, sense and identify each part of your musculature and skeletal structure. It is impossible to practice them on your own; you are told at the beginning of the course that you must come to lessons at least four or five times per week. The movements are slow and gentle, and its advocates and practitioners insist on their effectiveness. They are based on gravity and structure, and a wealth of physical and mental benefits are attributed to them. Again, I am not going to argue with the devotees, but I found them to be the dullest exercises I have ever tried.

And now we come to *Rolfing*—an Esalen baby—and you are

just not anybody who is anybody if you haven't been Rolfed. Also called "Structural Integration," the theory is based on the body's relationship to gravity. Any childhood fall or accident is supposed to result in muscular trauma and the misalignment of your body and mind. Through Rolfing you release physical and mental trauma and tension, effecting favorable changes in your basic structural system and in the chemistry of your body. Its originator is Dr. Ida Rolf, a biochemist who taught her method to very few. I truly thought myself to be an ideal candidate for Rolfing, for I had suffered a severe accident which threw every part of my structure out of kilter, and my posture was nothing to shout about. I found a Rolfer who claimed to be an M.D. The course consists of ten sessions in which the Rolfer works on the myofasciae, the tissues that envelop and support the muscles. He digs into your body with his fingers, fists, arms, elbows and feet—every single part of your body, including your eyes and the roof of your mouth. I have a high threshold of pain, and I used Yoga breathing to lessen the pain, but let me tell you that it was the most excruciating ordeal I have ever suffered voluntarily. After each session the Rolfer went into ecstasies about how greatly my posture had improved. The Rolfee felt and saw nothing. I suffered through all ten sessions and did not experience one iota of improvement. My pocketbook suffered as well, because the course was extremely expensive. I am sure that Dr. Rolf is sincere, but for me Rolfing did not work.

In the same category as the aforementioned fall William Reich's Orgonomic Therapy, Bioenergenetics, Centering, and many, many more.

While the body boom is flourishing, the mind-improvement, mind-expansion and consciousness-raising activities for sale have cornered today's market. Our stress-and-strain society is searching frantically for any relief from tension, for the peace of mind and mental fitness needed to deal with everyday life. The road of evolution is toward self-improvement, but someone or something is desperately needed to show us the way, and where there's demand, there is supply. There is a fortune to be made in the self-improvement field. All that is needed is a gimmick and the funds to promote and advertise it; if it promises relief from tension, personality change, restoration of self-confidence, or psychic powers, it will be bought.

So we have TM and T.A., Arica and est, Scientology, Mind Dynamics, Silva's Mind Control, Eckankar, Psychic Development; and more are springing up each day. People are traveling from one mind-blowing thing to another, looking for the answer of life. The lingo differs, as each method seems to develop a vocabulary of its own. In Scientology it's "engrams"; in Arica, "chinch" and "mentation." Silva's Mind Control slogans are "cancel—cancel" and "right-on," and est specializes in four-letter words. All these methods are contrivances, a mishmash of religions, Freud, Dale Carnegie, Encounter (Whatever happened to "Encounter"?), Zen and, most of all, Yoga. Some employ Yoga exercises and breathing, and all use Yoga relaxation techniques. Some of these courses I have taken, some of the methods I have tried and discarded, and some of them are on my shopping list. All methods have this in common: whatever course or workshop you sign up for, you have to pay in advance. The costs range from moderate to excessive. They uniformly employ brainwashing, programming, auto-conditioning and hypnotism. For two days or four days, or two weekends or six weeks, or whatever, you are told over and over again (a) that you are smart, great, a genius; that you have psychic and healing powers; and (b) that this particular system is the only one that can make you realize and use your potential. You believe these things gladly and are happy that you got your money's worth, especially if the course works, and in most cases it does. On the "plus" side there is really nothing wrong or unethical about any of the methods I have mentioned. The concepts and moral attitudes are good, and many people are helped, especially those who arrive via the drug or alcohol scene. But unfortunately some of the seekers are mentally unbalanced, and when they are led into trances or outer-space trips by psychiatrically untrained personnel, their disturbances frequently become magnified, and bad things can happen. For the average person who has not been exposed to anything else and who has not experienced the full effects of Yoga practice, I can well understand how some of these methods are like new doors opening up. I try to explore everything with an open mind, always hoping to learn a new method or technique to enrich my teaching of Yoga, and very often I do. There is a bit of truth in everything, but the point I am trying to make is that you must not accept one person's "proven" method as the ultimate opinion or one person's brainchild as the absolute truth. Not even Einstein or Freud proved to be infallible. And this is where Yoga comes in. It is not one course, technique or method. It is not a one-time undertaking which you pay for, apply and eventually shelve. Yoga is the science of life and the art of living. It is the commonsense answer to overall physical and mental fitness. In Yoga you will find all the physical movements that you need for superb overall physical health, and all the relaxation and meditation techniques to assure mental fitness and health, with a minimum of time, effort and expense.

All methods work if you apply them. It is not the method but the self-discipline and everyday practice of whatever you have learned that bring the desired results. Someone or something may lead you along the way, but no one can be with you all the time, and ultimately you yourself have to take over. The key to lifelong fitness is to establish a program that is feasible to incorporate into your life and to do every day. It must be uncomplicated, must take only a minimum of time, and must require no gadgets, special equipment, instructor, or manipulator at your side. It must be fun to do, and it must bring progressively evident results for it to work. There are, of course, those disciplinarians who religiously do two hundred pushups or one hour of strenuous calisthenics every day, not because they enjoy it, but because they believe it to be good for them. These are the minority. I am addressing myself to the average sedentary and rather lazy American who realizes the necessity to be fit but wants it to blend into his general life style. None of the above-mentioned exercise programs fill the requirement, because all are geared to sporadic rather than steady and lasting fitness.

Yoga, however, can easily be incorporated into one's life style. The only equipment needed is a towel, and very little space is required. I travel quite a bit and have managed to practice in the smallest of hotel rooms. About two years ago there was a newspaper article by a reporter who had been imprisoned in China. He practiced Yoga in his cell and held on to his sanity, optimism and health. It is impossible to remember a great variety of movements, but in Yoga you need only three or four basic movements to keep you in optimum fitness. It is the everyday repetition that brings the desired results, and I will elaborate on this matter later on in the book. Anyone, no matter how busy, can spend ten minutes a day on exercises, five minutes on breathing and fifteen minutes to a half-hour on meditation. In a few weeks' time you will discover that this can make the difference between feeling blah and feeling great every day of your life.

Many people do not realize that Yoga is an exercise. They equate Yoga positions, especially the more acrobatic ones, with an Indian self-torture system on a par with sleeping on nails or walking on glass. The fact is that Yoga is the most superb exercise system ever devised. The exercises are based on natural movements of the body and are for everyone from eight to eighty. There is no other exercise system that reaches every part of the musculoskeletal systems, no other method that exercises the inner organs as well as the outer body. In order for the body to be in perfect physical condition, every single part of it must be used.

There is much emphasis today on cardiovascular health. But the heart muscle is only one of the 636 muscles in the body. A strong, healthy heart is of great importance, but it is not indicative of general overall health. The detractors of Yoga point out that all Yoga movements are slow and that they do not activate the heart muscle. This is quite untrue, because there are a number of Yoga movements and positions (Sun Salutation, Cobra, Locust, Bow) which greatly accelerate the heartbeat and pulse rate. Leading cardiologists agree that a worthwhile exercise program should incorporate movements that involve flexion, extension and rotation of the entire body. Every position of Yoga incorporates these movements; Yoga is designed to promote complete flexibility of the entire musculoskeletal system. Also, leading cardiologists and physical-fitness experts feel that any good program of physical fitness must develop strength, skill and endurance. Through the movements of Yoga, if they are practiced consistently, these will be developed.

In fast-moving exercise, muscles are bunched, jerked, bobbed and bounced, and thereby foreshortened. Forceful contractions and extensions develop muscle mass through the tightening and shortening of the muscles. In Yoga the muscles are slowly stretched, elongated and elasticized, rather than being trained to snap back like a rubberband. They stay stretched and resilient.

Skeletal deterioration is associated with aging. Recent medical findings relate this to a decrease in muscle mass and indicate that everyday stretching of the muscles will help prevent deterioration of the bone. It is a fact that the rigid musculature caused by standard exercise programs depletes energy, whereas a flexible, supple body and mind release energy, so that one can fulfill one's highest human potential.

Yoga exercises and breathing techniques, correctly and consistently performed, relax the body as well as the mind. By stretching the body to relieve physical tension, we release mental tension as well. Physical fitness leads to mental fitness, and no other mind-expanding program is needed.

2

YOGA
AND
ME

MY PERSONAL PHILOSOPHY regarding the flow of life is that roughly seventy-five percent is self-controlled and twenty-five percent is in the hands of some uncontrollable force—destiny, karma, cosmic intelligence, God, or whatever you want to call it. Obviously I stumbled into Yoga by chance, but I believe that the chain of events that led me to Yoga was predestined.

I was born in Berlin into a middle-class, very proper and staid German Jewish family. I went through all the trials and tribulations of growing up, but had a more or less normal childhood and led a very protected and sheltered life. There was no premonition that it would not always be so and no doubt that I would grow up in Germany in my parents' home, go to school, get married, and so on. I was spoiled, used to getting my own way, and completely unprepared to cope with life.

A phenomenon called Hitler destroyed and changed millions of lives, including mine, and on the brink of war my father whisked me out of Germany and brought me to live with distant relatives in California. He unfortunately returned to Germany, but a year later he managed to have my brother join me. During the next few years I moved from family to family, going to school, working, and, I must confess, feeling pretty sorry for myself. Then at last, as the gates of Europe had almost slammed shut for Jews, my mother managed to get out and dock in New York. Overjoyed, I joined her there as soon as I could. My father later died in a concentration camp.

After the war I returned to Europe. By now I was an American citizen working as an interpreter for the United States Army, first in France and then in Germany. In Germany I met Eric, who had fought in the Danish underground against the Nazis and was now also working for the American Army. We fell in love, but, as Army employees, found ourselves wound in red tape when we wanted to get married.

The days before our wedding were spent filling out countless forms and wrestling with Army regulations complicating our intentions. In the end love—and perseverance—did triumph. The red tape was cut, and we were married under official sanction of the United States Army. The bride wore khaki. So did the groom.

Not long after that the Army agencies in Germany were dissolved, and we found ourselves out of jobs. Enjoying ourselves too much to leave the party, we decided to remain in Europe awhile before returning to the States. We gypsied through Europe, starting various businesses, only to have them fail because of our own inexperience, bad luck, or a combination of both. We lived in Israel four years before finally returning to the United States, with empty pockets but not empty hands, because by then we had a four-year-old daughter, Carolyn.

Once we were back in New York, my husband found a job, we signed a lease on an apartment, and I became pregnant again. The only thing missing was money. To help out, I got a job. Every weekend, when my husband was home to take care of our daughter, I packed up and went to work at one of the large luxury resorts in the nearby Catskill Mountains. I received my salary, board, and room in a ramshackle firetrap reserved for the hotel's help.

One winter night, as the staff lay sleeping, fire broke out. I was in a room on the third floor, and like many others I was trapped by spreading flames consuming the single wooden staircase and cutting off escape. Screams of "Fire! Fire!" reached me as in a dream. Exhausted, I snuggled down deeper into my bed, wanting—strangely enough—nothing so much as to stay right where I was. Indeed, having faced death then and also at other times, let me assure those who dread it that death is not that terrifying when you are confronted with it. What saved me were my instincts rather than my intellect. Without really thinking out my actions, I got up and looked around for a way to escape. There was only one possible means—the two windows in this third-floor dormitory. One window was always stuck closed. The other was open but blocked by the other occupants trying to escape the fast-approaching flames. I smashed through the stuck window and crawled out onto the ledge. I strained to hear the sound of an approaching fire engine through the cold night, but there was none. When the flames came unbearably close, I let go, plummeting down to the concrete-covered ground. By the time the fire engine did arrive, the building had burned to the ground and ten people were dead. I am convinced that if these people had relied on their common sense they would not have died. Later, when those of us who had survived discussed the fire, we all agreed that because of the shock and the sudden disturbance of sleep we had reacted instinctively, almost like sleepwalkers.

The bodies of those who died revealed that they were so bound by dogmas of convention and propriety that they obviously couldn't use their instinctive common sense. Some of the victims had wasted valuable time by putting on underwear and stockings because of modesty, or by going back for their possessions. Others could think only of trying to escape by the stairs, which had already become impassable. Those of us who had immediately followed our instincts and jumped were injured, some crippled for life, *but all had survived.*

Unrestricted common sense proved to be the difference between life and death. Obviously there are other times in life when consequences will not be so final, yet to enable ourselves to really live in the fullest meaning of the word we must break the chains that bind our common sense.

As a result of the jump, I suffered a fractured spine, broken pelvic and pubic bones, and internal injuries—and, among those who had jumped from the third floor, I was one of the lucky ones. But of course I lost my unborn baby.

The fire and its immediate results were a nightmare to live through. Now, many years later, I can look back on it philosophically, without anguish, and tell about it as any other experience, not only because it happened a long time ago, but because I strongly believe that it was necessary for me to have lived that tragedy in order to have a keener appreciation of my present happiness. Also, that fire was a milestone in my life because it brought me to Yoga.

Fortunately, workmen's compensation shouldered the burden of my medical expenses and the cost of the various contraptions my body was confined within. For starters, I spent two months in the hospital encased in a back cast. When that came off, I was released and locked into a steel brace. Ultimately, I graduated to various steel-enforced corsets which I was told I would have to wear for the rest of my life. Even taking a few steps without my corset meant subjecting myself to excruciating pain. As an outpatient at one of the finest rehabilitation hospitals in the country, I underwent a series of massages, heat treatments, and stretchings. My injuries had mended, but the pain persisted. I was a physical and mental wreck, although compared to the other patients in that hospital I could have been classified 1-A. I walked through the hospital door on my own two feet, while almost all the other patients rode in wheelchairs, some without arms or legs, others merely torsos. But I was feeling far too sorry for myself to have any sympathy for anyone else. Most of the staff were also disabled. In particular, I remember the crippled social worker, a remarkable woman with a great feeling of compassion for me. Although she sat in a wheelchair to interview me, I envied her, because I could sense she possessed what I lacked—peace of mind. During the course of treatment, psychological therapy had been advised, but my husband couldn't pay for that, and the insurance company had refused to pay the expenses. By sheer tenacity, this woman arranged for psychotherapy sessions for me and somehow persuaded the compensation board to pay for them. Now I only want to mention that psychotherapy helped me to hang on. Later, I will explain more about Yoga's relation to psychiatry. Eventually, I was laced into my final corset and sent out into the world to "resume a normal life." At that time, my normal life meant, in addition to the strictures of the corset, continuous pain, overweight, fatigue, nervousness, insomnia, and three packs of cigarettes daily. In short, I was a mess. However, I must give myself credit for one good quality, at least—I was a fighter, even if I usually fought in the wrong direction. For instance, during my better periods I looked for work and took jobs, which I usually couldn't handle. I went to school and took the wrong courses, joined organizations which bored me to death, and even tried physical programs which left me frustrated and in tears. There were times I was so desperate that I started looking for different religions to convert to, but before I took any steps, my common sense managed to make itself heard by firmly saying, "No." My only successful venture was to give birth to our second daughter, Judy. I managed to pull myself together for that event, but shortly thereafter I fell apart again.

A friend of mine who had been in the fire and who also jumped had suffered a back injury more serious than mine. She had been in and out of a cast for many years without results. Finally she underwent the spinal fusion which had been put off as the last resort because of the seriousness of the operation. Fortunately, it was successful. A few days after she left the hospital, I went to see her. Naturally, I was outfitted in my corset, which incidentally added to my girth and detracted from my self-confidence, and expected my friend to be similarly supported. But, to my amazement, she was wearing absolutely no support whatsoever. Considering myself an authority in the proper care and treatment of back injuries, I was curious as to why her doctor had not prescribed a brace. "Because," she answered, "he claims that my back muscles would not have a chance to regain their strength naturally." The obvious common sense of this was like a revelation. My own bones and muscles had healed but had never been given the opportunity to regain their strength. Artificially constricted for years by braces and corsets, they were incapable of holding up on their own; in the ensuing years I have observed and concluded that restricting garments in general are a health hazard. The Victorian ladies who had to be saddled into their stays may have had tiny waists, but they also had short, sick lives. Western women, aghast at the old Chinese custom of binding girls' feet, have probably done more harm to their own internal organs with corsets. Corsets and girdles compress vital organs, muscles, and tissues and impair circulation. At present the trend is toward more natural unconstricting underwear. But one never knows what new body shape will be hailed next as the epitome of beauty, and millions of women will squeeze their bodies into bone, steel, and plastic in an effort to achieve it. (It has been proved that the truss, for years the standard accessory for hernia cases, does more damage than good.) If my muscles had been weakened by lack of use, I reasoned, they could be strengthened by use. In other words, what my sluggish back muscles needed was exercise. It seems incredible now that not one doctor among the many that I consulted, not even those at the rehabilitation center, had ever suggested exercise. To me exercise meant calisthenics. With new-found enthusiasm I joined a gym and started the 1-2-3-4, up and down, left and right routine—and then collapsed in pain. Realizing the need for guidance, I went to the sensible doctor who had operated on my friend. He agreed that I was on the right track, but on the wrong exercise, and gave me a set of exercises of his own invention. They were quite dull, most of them were done pressing against a wall. Hopefully, I practiced religiously for a few months, varying the walls I pressed against in an attempt to inject some interest into the exercises. They did me no harm, as calisthenics had, but I couldn't detect any improvement.

Discouraged, but still open to suggestions, I listened with interest to one of those thirdhand stories about a friend of a friend of a friend who had benefited greatly from Yoga exercises. "Why not Yoga?" I asked myself. After all, I had tried everything else. And I ventured forth to find a teacher.

Although Yoga was already popular on the West Coast, at

that time it was literally unheard of in New York and often confused with yogurt, Yogi Bear, and Yogi Berra. Under "Yoga" in the Manhattan phone directory there was little choice. I came up with a book store, a disconnected number, a Yogi who, I was told, was presently in India, and one person who answered and said, yes, he was a teacher and available for private lessons. I made an appointment, bringing a friend with me for protection because I vaguely associated Yoga with opium dens and white slavery. Contrary to my expectations, I found a pleasant-looking Indian in Western dress. He cast a sympathetic eye at my lumpy figure and suggested we give Yoga exercises a try.

When I first began my weekly lessons, my situation seemed as hopeless as teaching Yoga to an oak tree, for I could not bend in any direction. My stubborn muscles resisted the new demands being made on them. But as the weeks went by I loosened up more and more. After three months I threw away my corset. Since that day I have worn no support of any kind, and my back has become stronger than it has ever been. I had gone into Yoga for the limited purpose of strengthening my back. Having accomplished that, after a year I discarded Yoga. I was convinced that Yoga was superior to any other kind of exercise, but I was completely ignorant of its full meaning. I did not backslide into all my pre-Yoga ways. I cherished my new limberness and at times even practiced, especially the Headstand, which had taken me so long to master. Life seemed to take a turn for the better, although, except for my new flexibility, I appeared much the same. I was still overweight, nervous, tired, and smoking three packs of cigarettes daily. In spite of all this, I was happier with myself in my role as wife and mother, and my family was happy with me.

As far as I was concerned, Yoga had had all the impact on my life it was ever going to have—but I was mistaken. As I mentioned, I was overweight and, not surprisingly, so was my younger daughter. In fact, my husband and I both come from a long line of what anxious mothers call good eaters, and our whole family is inclined toward obesity. My daughter has been a roly-poly from the day she was born. Besides constantly watching her diet, I had always been on the lookout for physical activities for her. Meanwhile, California Yoga teachers had begun to infiltrate New York, and, although not yet exactly a household word, Yoga became a little better known. By chance I heard about a mother-daughter Yoga program in which I enthusiastically enrolled myself and my reluctant younger daughter Judy. After a few lessons, daughter became a Yoga dropout. But mother remained because (a) I had paid for the course in advance, (b) I found that working with a class was fun, and (c) I suddenly caught a glimpse of a more hopeful future.

After completing that course, I reenrolled and progressed from intermediate student to advanced. By this time I was quite interested in Yoga—I even signed up for a teacher-training course—although the possibility of my teaching Yoga was the furthest thing from my mind. But day by day, as I demonstrated exercises in front of the class with ever-growing confidence, I realized that here was something that I could do well and help other people by doing. Gradually I began to accept the fact that there was nothing in the world that I wanted more than to become a Yoga teacher. And I, who had never really directed my energies toward achieving any goal, suddenly knew how to go about it—by applying myself with discipline and hard work. In the past I had always worked belligerently, but now I worked with a slow, steady deliberation born of my purpose of mind. I knew that consistency was the vital factor in achieving my goal. I don't mean that I turned my whole day over to Yoga, because after all I still had my family to care for, but I practiced conscientiously one hour a day. I never exceeded an hour of practice, because to overdo it would have defeated my purpose. Through sheer mechanical practice, everything fell into line. My figure improved. I was healthier and more energetic. For the first time in years I fell asleep easily. I gradually eliminated tranquilizers and barbiturates, which up to that time had been a staple part of my diet. Quite naturally and painlessly I gave up smoking.

As my body changed, my mental outlook and attitude did also. It was nothing drastic or sudden, but a slow manifestation of character change. My sense of values became different, and so did my attitude toward people. I developed more patience, kindness, tolerance, and compassion. At the same time, I was better able to stand up to those who browbeat me and tried to impose their values on me. Developing a great hunger for knowledge of all kinds, I felt a whole new world of learning opening up for me.

For financial reasons I had had to leave college shortly after starting, and through the years I had blamed that fact not only for my lack of knowledge, but also for many of my other inadequacies. One of the greatest frustrations of my life was the failure to have a satisfying career. But instead of doing something about it, I had daydreamed, mostly about being a teacher of some kind because I had always felt that I had something to offer in this world. Now I knew that I was meant to teach Yoga, to pass on the benefits that I had received to as many people as possible.

I read all the Yoga books ever written. I sought out many teachers in order to learn as much as I could about all phases of Yoga. As I searched, I found quite a variety of Yoga teachers, some good, some bad, some indifferent, but I was able to learn something from each of them. Then I simply started to teach. The more I taught, the more I learned, and I will never stop learning. Reaping more and more benefits through Yoga, I gradually felt the limits of what I could achieve melt away. For the first time in my life I experienced satisfaction and confidence in my work. I knew that this was only the beginning. I could attain my goals because now I knew which route to take. My greatest goal was to inform as many people as possible about Yoga. I don't believe in pressuring anyone to take up Yoga, but those who are searching for a way to give meaning to their lives should know how to find it. I am aware, on the other hand, that too many people have misconceptions about Yoga and therefore hesitate to enrich their lives through it. Every day, wherever I go, I see someone to whom I'd like to say, "Be sensible. Yoga is for you." That is why I have written this book.

3

YOGA:
ITS MEANING
AND
TRADITION

MOST PEOPLE no longer think of Yoga as preparation for lying on a bed of nails. However, there is still a great deal of confusion over what Yoga actually is. Basically, Yoga is a system of physical and mental self-improvement that people have been using for thousands of years. Its beginnings have been traced back to the Upanishads and Bhagavad Gita, both part of the ancient Sanskrit epic of Hindu philosophy called the Vedas. The Bhagavad Gita, perhaps the most quoted of all Hindu literature, is considered by some the Yogic bible. Around the second century B.C. the basic principles and practices of Yoga were set down in the Yoga Sutras by Patanjali, who is sometimes called the Father of Yoga.

All these works were written in Sanskrit, an ancient language that is extremely difficult to translate and therefore open to a broad range of interpretation. Indeed, it is possible that ten different Sanskrit scholars will come up with ten different meanings for the same word. Realizing this, it is easy to understand why, although the basic Yoga principles have been preserved, there now exists a wide variety of applications. Consequently, there have arisen a multitude of Yoga societies and schools of thought, each with its own particular advocate, each claiming to possess the true Yoga. I sincerely believe that what I teach, commonsense Yoga, is true Yoga. It follows the classic rules of an ancient wisdom, philosophy, and science but custom-tailors them for practical application to the needs of twentieth-century Western civilization. Most importantly, it works effectively for me and my students.

I have gathered knowledge from all the Yoga teachers I have studied with and all the Yoga books I have read, but I have placed none on a pedestal as the ultimate authority. The true meaning of Yoga I find within myself, as you will, learning what is natural and right for you. In effect, the mark of common sense is having this ability to choose from many opinions what is best for you. People who cannot do this spend their lives floundering in a hopeless quandary. As an example, I have an acquaintance who raises her children by the book. By book, I mean the profusion of books written on child behavior. She reads them all. Not only does each author have a different opinion on child rearing, but the pendulum of child psychology is constantly swinging between the extremes of discipline and permissiveness. One year it's "Spank the child," another "Don't lay a hand on him." My friend is continually applying every new theory that appears on the horizon, with the result that her children, who started life as normal human beings, have now been turned into neurotics.

While adapting Yoga to our present-day needs, I do not compromise its name and tradition. For instance, once when I applied to teach at a religious institution, I was granted permission, but with the stipulation that I call my course "Yogamatics," or some other phony title, to appease the religious leader, who thought that Yoga was a religion. The course never materialized. Yoga is Yoga.

There are certain terms and ideas that will add significance and beauty to your initiation into Yoga. On the other hand, I am avoiding the complexities of Yoga philosophy and the use of tongue-twisting Sanskrit terms to describe the various postures, for at this stage they would serve no purpose in successful practice.

Yoga, most simply interpreted, means union, the union of the body, mind, and spirit. There are many Yogas: Hatha, Raja, Jnana, Bhakti, Karma, and Mantra, to name but a few. The ultimate goal of all these Yogas is the same—the supreme realization of self. I have chosen to concentrate on and teach only Hatha and Raja Yoga, because with a sensible amount of time and effort, these most adequately fulfill our needs.

Hatha Yoga

Hatha is the Yoga of physical culture, combining body-stretching postures and regulated breathing, designed to produce the utmost flexibility, health, and vitality. The word "Hatha" comes from the Sanskrit words "Ha," meaning sun, and "Tha," meaning moon. It refers to the balance of these two forces, corresponding to the positive and negative forces in the body.

Calisthenics, rhythm exercises, isometrics, and dance movements are all incorporated into Hatha Yoga and, in fact, partially originated from it. Pioneers of modern dance studied Yoga and used its positions as the basis for developing their dance movements. Yoga has no quick or jerky movements. All its exercises are executed slowly, gracefully, and thoughtfully, without straining. With Yoga you aren't expected to huff and puff to get results, which is why it is the ideal exercise for any age group.

There are the classic postures, or *asanas*, often patterned after movements of different animals, and, in addition, numerous other exercises which have been developed by various Yoga teachers. Actually, any calisthenic or dance movement can become a Yoga position by being held static with proper breath control, for that is the key to Yoga practice. Almost all Yoga positions are held for a period of time in order to receive the maximum benefit from each exercise. This is one of the many reasons why Yoga is superior to other forms of exercise. By remaining motionless, we allow the body to stretch naturally to its own capacity.

All we do is maintain the posture without forcing and let the body do the work of stretching unused muscles, ligaments, and tendons. This stretching and holding to our own individual capacity is what firms our muscles, makes our body more flexible, and builds up our physical endurance. As most people begin Yoga with a stiff, inflexible body, they experience an initial discomfort which soon disappears. Remember, this discomfort is natural after putting rarely used muscles to work. Rushing into an exercise can cause damage, but no damage can be done by the gradual deliberateness of Yoga, which requires no more of your body than it is able to accomplish. You'll be surprised how much your body will be able to accomplish with consistent Yoga practice.

The other vital aspect of Hatha Yoga is regulated breathing. We can live without food or water for surprisingly long periods of time, but deprive us of breath for a few moments and we die. Considering this, it is amazing how little attention is given to proper breathing.

Breathing is virtually ignored by physical educators as a prerequisite of health and by medical authorities as a preventive of disease; however, I notice that in certain areas breathing is coming into its own. When respiratory illness becomes acute, as in cases of asthma, bronchitis, or emphysema, patients are often introduced to proper breathing. Also, there are advocates of natural childbirth who teach Yoga breathing to pregnant women to achieve relaxation of the pelvic muscles and nervous system during labor and childbirth. Some psychiatrists instruct patients in proper breathing to induce calmness. Unfortunately, other than these patients, it seems that only opera singers and method actors have been singled out to receive training in how to breathe. We're told often enough to get out in the open and take a really deep breath. But once there we're left hanging because no one has ever told us what to do with that breath and where to put it. Does it seem strange that it should be necessary to teach something as natural as breathing? Well, chances are we would not do something as natural as walking upright if we were not taught. A child raised by four-legged creatures probably would never straighten its body, but rather would walk on all fours. Or if a child were brought up in a mute society, he would never learn to speak. Some functions are intrinsic to man; others must be acquired. Correct breathing is one of the latter.

Yoga teaches us to breathe slowly and deeply to the fullest capacity of our lungs, filtering and purifying our breath by breathing through the nose. Obviously, the deeper we breathe, the more air we inhale, the more oxygen our body receives. A greater amount of oxygen reaching the heart means a healthier and more efficient heart and entire cardiovascular system. As we breathe more deeply, we must necessarily breathe more slowly, decreasing tension and increasing serenity: important factors to consider with the ever growing concern with heart disease. In addition, the blood is purified, resulting in a healthy skin and glowing complexion. Complete Yoga breathing also ensures an increased supply of oxygen to the brain, thus increasing mental alertness and clarity. In a society plagued by minor respiratory disorders, as evidenced by the countless products promising to relieve them, Yoga breathing offers a genuine method of attaining a healthy respiratory system. By bringing oxygen to the whole lung, the walls of the lung are cleansed of poisonous particles that are inhaled—certainly important these days when experts are warning that smoking and the pollution level of our air have reached dangerous proportions.

The list of Yoga breathing exercises is practically endless, but it is neither feasible nor necessary to practice most of them. Through experimentation, I have limited the breathing exercises to those easiest to adopt and most potent when perfected.

Marvelous as the results of Hatha Yoga are, most Eastern teachings stick Hatha Yoga on the bottom rung of the Yogic ladder, conceding that the body should be in perfect shape, but only as a step toward perfecting the spiritual state. The Hindu in general, including certain sects of Yogis, is less concerned with the body, except as an adjunct to the spirit, because of his belief in reincarnation. He considers his body only a temporary abode for his spirit, which, to him, is far more real than his body. The soul, or self, is a complete entity, distinct from the body, experiencing neither birth nor death, but inhabiting different physical forms at different times, in a series of reincarnations.

The belief in reincarnation, in being reborn into a new body, which is so prevalent in Eastern philosophy, is rejected by most Western minds. Yet there is no definitive disproof of it, and I would like you to at least open your mind to the possibility that life may continue in different forms.

There are many cases on record of people who knew things they could not have learned in their present lives, and although skeptics have tried to refute their claims to past lives, the tantalizing possibility remains.

To the believer, reincarnation provides the answer to the

age-old questions man has always asked regarding injustice and undeserved suffering in the world, for whatever man suffers in this life is his just punishment for his sins in his previous life. Because man's life is determined by his actions in his past life, the tragedies and inequalities that befall him are solely of his own doing. If his present life is righteous, he will be rewarded in his next life.

In this ongoing cycle of birth, death, and rebirth, one can see how the emphasis must be placed on the soul rather than the body. The more the soul can separate itself from the body, the greater the bliss it will experience. Yoga is the means used to liberate the soul from the body. When the soul is completely liberated and reunited with the universal soul, it will have been freed once and for all from its bondage to the physical world.

However, as non-ascetic, practical Westerners, we are not striving for what the Easterner considers spiritual purification. Hatha Yoga is not merely the way toward achievement; it is itself the achievement. Our goal is the attainment of a healthy, youthful, relaxed body through the practice of Hatha Yoga. This, in turn, can lead us to peace of mind, because the body and the mind are one, completely interdependent. Controlling and relaxing the body through Hatha Yoga will eventually lead into Raja Yoga, the Yoga of meditation. In Chapter 6, I will discuss this method of disciplining the mind toward the path of self-realization. Now I would like to give you a brief idea of some of the other important Yogas.

Jnana Yoga

Jnana Yoga is the Yoga of the intellect, considered to be the most difficult of all Yogas, to be undertaken and mastered only by those who have achieved purity of thought by practicing the other Yogas. The sensory world and all knowledge received through the senses are considered an illusion. True knowledge, that is, knowledge of the soul, is sought through intellectual analysis. Past, present, and future are interwoven into timeless existence. The concept of "I" becomes meaningless. The individual self is liberated by merging with the universal Self, pure spirit, or Atman.

Bhakti Yoga

In contrast to Jnana Yoga, Bhakti Yoga seeks salvation through love. It is the devotional Yoga, offering a much more direct approach to spiritual fulfillment in this world. It resembles the practices of Western religions but requires no house of worship. The follower of Bhakti Yoga prays to God, Brahman, or Hindu deities either alone, at home, or in ceremonies with a spiritual leader. Bhakti Yoga is actually the only Yoga with which the majority of Indians are familiar.

Karma Yoga

This is the Yoga of action. The ideal of the Karma Yogi is work for the work's sake and not for the fruit of his work. Freed from desire and attachment to worldly things, he finds spiritual liberation in pure action. He alone is responsible for his actions, and through his actions he shapes his destiny, present and future. Karma Yoga appeals most to the Westerner because it emphasizes self-realization through action.

Mantra Yoga

Mantra Yoga is the Yoga of sound and vibration. Mantras are sacred syllables used in prayer or meditation. They are repeated silently or aloud in chants or incantations. It is said that each Mantra possesses a certain psychic energy and that indefinite repetition of a Mantra endows the individual with psychic powers. It is customary for a Swami* or Guru to choose a special Mantra to benefit each person, according to the message he receives from the individual's vibrations. The Mantra is usually a salutation to a Hindu luminary, such as "Hare Krishna" (Hail Krishna). The secret of the Mantra is zealously guarded and must never be revealed to another person.

The boundaries between these different Yogas are not always sharp and distinct. Very often their principles and practices overlap. Basic to all Yoga is the idea of *Prana*, the life force. Essential to life, it is found in every living thing, from the most elementary form of plant life to the most complex form of animal life. It is in matter, but it is not matter. It is in the air, but it is not air. It is inhaled along with oxygen, but it is not oxygen. Too subtle to be graphically pinpointed, Prana exists as surely as do electricity and cosmic rays. Its abstract quality is comparable to that of what is termed "the soul." The soul is commonly accepted as a spiritual part of every individual, although it cannot be seen. In the same way, we can understand the existence of Prana.

Writings of the ancient Hebrews and Greeks referred to Prana, but it is not found in more modern Western writings. Perhaps the closest we can come to the conception of Prana is vitality. This special vitality reveals itself as a definite element of our physical and mental constitution to all who seriously practice Yoga. Even the most down-to-earth practitioner will come to accept the existence of Prana. I, who at

---

*The titles "Swami," "Guru," and "Yogi" cause a great deal of confusion, and understandably so, for they're often used interchangeably. *Guru* is simply the Sanskrit word for teacher. A person who practices Yoga can be called a *Yogi, Yogin*, or, if female, *Yogini*. A *Swami* is an adherent of a spiritual order following the teachings of a particular Hindu saint or luminary; both men and women can become Swamis—most vow celibacy. The title is bestowed by another Swami, usually the teacher, together with the name of a departed saint and the ending "ananda," meaning bliss. Swami is also used in India as a form of address, meaning "Master," "Patron," or "Householder."

one time was only going through the motions of living and was actually "lifeless," have become "lifeful" through Yoga.

Prana is taken into the body, along with breath, by Pranayama or Yoga breathing, which I will explain further in the chapter on meditation. Once Prana has been absorbed and its presence felt, the utmost should be done to preserve it and prevent its being wasted. The advanced Yoga student learns to store Prana in the body by locking all the openings of his body. But there are more practical ways of preserving Prana, which even the beginner can carry out in the course of everyday life. These involve our thoughts and actions.

Every good and optimistic thought is an intake of Prana, just as an evil or pessimistic thought is a waste of Prana. The same applies to our actions—I'm not referring to standards set up by others, but what, in the ultimate analysis, constitutes what is good or bad for you. As Shakespeare said, "To thine own self be true." Many people would benefit if the Golden Rule were revised to: "Do unto yourself what you would do unto others." In other words, please yourself before you please others, for the very good reason that you cannot truly benefit others unless you are happy with yourself. When you act without regard to your own satisfaction, you are dissipating your Prana.

We all have duties and obligations that we must fulfill. However, many people take on additional jobs or duties— chairman of the PTA or a hospital volunteer—because they think they should or the community expects it. Now, if you love pounding the gavel for the PTA or working with the sick, there could be no better way to utilize your spare time. On the other hand, if you suffer through the meetings in utter boredom or can't stand the sight of blood, you are defeating your own purpose of wanting to do good, and you are wasting your Prana. Another waste of Prana is meaningless action, such as tapping your feet, chewing on a pencil, or doodling.

Then there are certain people who will drain your reservoir

of Prana if you let them. Unfortunately, sometimes you have to cope with these people, if, for instance, one of them happens to be your boss or mother-in-law. But we all have acquaintances, very often neighbors, who bore and agitate us, who we wish would vanish from our lives, but whom we put up with, because we feel we should. I'm not suggesting that you insult them, throw them out bodily, or tell them off—which, by the way, does the least good—but you should make a decided effort to detach yourself from these people who are sapping your vitality. Keep this in mind in the beginning of Yoga practice. Later, after you have increased your store of Prana and gained serenity through Yoga, you will be better able to deal with these people. Seek out and associate with those who radiate vitality, whose presence stimulates and refreshes you.

The Yogi believes that Pranic energy is preserved throughout the body in storage centers called *Chakras*—literally translated, circles or wheels. Each Chakra has a lotus flower attached. These subtle centers of consciousness are located along the spine. The six basic Chakras are at the base of the spine, at the genitals, near the navel, near the heart, near the throat, and between the eyebrows. In a category by itself is the Chakra at the top of the brain containing a thousand-petaled lotus. The ancient legendary scheme of Chakras was, no doubt, the forerunner of what is now called the autonomic nervous system, the involuntary regulator of the body.

The third Chakra is the solar plexus, referred to as the abdominal brain both by the Yogi and by modern science. It is a nerve center of the sympathetic nervous system that branches out to and regulates all the abdominal viscera. Less than a hundred years ago the solar plexus gained a certain notoriety when boxing champion James Corbett was knocked out by a well-landed punch to his solar plexus. Often, emotional reactions are described as a feeling in "the pit of the stomach" or "butterflies in the stomach."

The solar plexus is considered a major storage center of Prana from which the Yogi can draw strength, and even healing powers, to send into different directions. I'm sure that this is what has given rise to the misconception that the Yogi spends his time gazing upon his navel. The Yogi has no interest in his navel. It's the solar plexus, located behind the stomach, that he is concentrating upon when he sits and enters into meditation.

According to Yoga legend, by intensive concentration on Chakras the Yogi awakens *Kundalini,* the coiled serpent sleeping at the base of the spine. Kundalini can be translated as spiritual energy or basic power. The intricate processes involved in arousing Kundalini constitute a whole separate Yoga whereby the female Kundalini (a name I love to pronounce merely for the esthetic pleasure of its sound) is symbolically united with the male deity *Shiva.* Meditation on the six basic Chakras, beginning with the lowest one and moving upward, forces the Kundalini to move through a channel along the spinal cord. As she reaches each Chakra, its lotus petals open, pointing upward, until ultimately the thousand-petaled Chakra at the top of the brain is awakened. Piercing this final Chakra, the journey of Kundalini is completed and union with her spouse consummated.

There are many ways to interpret the Kundalini force. It represents the dormant elements in our personality, lying deep within our subconscious. Sexually, it is comparable to what Freud termed the libido, the sex urge, the psychic energy and force motivating human action, which, when released through psychoanalysis, reveals itself as the source of man's creative, emotional, and spiritual drives. Or you may call Kundalini the latent energy that you can learn to utilize through spiritual concentration and training. It can be thought of as basic intelligence, which is often blocked by negative thinking but which can be brought into the open by changing your ways of thinking. The awakening of Kundalini can also be compared to the realization of dreams and desires.

When the Kundalini bursts through the final Chakra, *Samadhi*, ecstasy, is achieved. Hindu legend says Samadhi can be experienced many times, ultimately resulting in *Nirvana*, which becomes the permanent state, with Kundalini and Shiva remaining united forever. Patanjali, however, considers the state of Samadhi to be the ultimate state. In Zen Buddhism *Satori* refers to the same experience.

The way to Samadhi is through the practice of Pranayama and meditation, according to the teachings of Patanjali. Samadhi is the state of superconsciousness, the greatest bliss. Here the highest truth, the mystery of life and death, is revealed. Some people mistakenly believe that Samadhi is a trance induced through meditation. There are many, as a matter of fact, who can easily enter into a trancelike state this way, but it is not Samadhi. On the contrary, Samadhi is a superawakening.

The Yogi holds that Samadhi is the prize for the one who has achieved complete spirituality, who has traded material desires for inner peace. It is the gateway to freedom of the soul. Broadly interpreted, Samadhi can be wisdom and maturity, the attainment of those virtues that lead to happiness, peace, and fulfillment.

Working toward Samadhi can be as meaningful as the achievement itself. I compare it to the striving of a truly great artist who all his life works toward perfection without regard to time.

The Japanese Sumi-e painter sometimes devotes his lifetime to the perfection of a single brush stroke. The great pianist Artur Rubinstein said, at the age of eighty-one, "Someday before I die, I hope to be able to play Beethoven's Fourth Symphony the way Beethoven would have wanted me to play it." This is not false modesty. It means that a true artist

never reaches that moment when he cries out, "I am perfect."
But by working toward perfection, he achieves much. Without actually attaining Samadhi, you can improve yourself and accomplish your goals. Therein lie peace and happiness.

4

YOGA:
WHAT IT
CAN DO
FOR YOU

Now you have an idea of what Yoga's all about. It's not some here today, gone tomorrow exercise fad. It's been bringing results for quite a while—for centuries, as a matter of fact. I will explain exactly how it will work for you.

Before people enroll in my course, they usually ask all kinds of questions about what Yoga can do for them. "Can it help me lose weight? Can it get rid of this potbelly? This dowager's hump? This spare tire? This dragged-out, tired look? This slump? Flab? Sag? Bulge? Droop?"

"Yes," I say. "Yes, Yoga can." But what they're really asking is, "Can Yoga make me look the way I want to look?" And how does everyone want to look? Beautiful, of course.

Beauty is many things. And pretty features alone don't

always add up to beauty. Granted, they help, but there are many beautiful women who possess eyes, a nose, and a mouth which are less than perfect. What *does* make a woman beautiful or a man handsome? A straight, firm body; a graceful way of moving; a poised, natural manner; smooth, glowing skin; a pleasant voice; and that sparkling aliveness that we call vitality. With these qualities a plain person can outshine someone more kindly endowed by nature. These are the very qualities that can be acquired by practicing Yoga exercises.

To the novice, the long list of benefits to be derived from Yoga may seem unbelievable. As you gain experience in Yoga, you will see that these promises can be confirmed by common sense. I can personally vouch for all the benefits I have listed, through both my own experience and the experiences of my students and other practitioners of Yoga I've known. My list would be even longer if I weren't disregarding those claims that I've only read or heard about. I'm sticking strictly to what I've seen.

Weight Control

Invariably beginners in Yoga ask, "Can I lose weight through Yoga exercises?" The only truthful answer is, "You can lose weight only through good eating habits." There is no other way. But if the question is, "Can Yoga *help* me to lose weight?" the answer is, "Most definitely, yes." Yoga exercises alone will not make the pounds roll off, but they will set off the weight loss and help the body maintain its proper weight. Most overeating is due to nervousness and tension. Many people will eat themselves into mountains when they are excited and agitated. People of different metabolism are affected the opposite way. Overly thin people are that way because when their nerves are on edge they can't eat, and the little food they do consume is worked off in nervous energy.

Yoga helps both these types of people. By practicing the exercises, breathing, and eventual meditation, you lose nervousness and stress, thereby eliminating the compulsion to either stuff or starve yourself.

It stands to reason that overweight is a great handicap to the successful practice of Hatha Yoga, but that does not mean that all thin people are limber and all heavy people inflexible. Many thin people are stiff as boards when they begin Yoga, and many overweight people move with agility. In general, of course, it is quite difficult to bend across a mountain of flesh when it's concentrated in the abdominal region, as is usually the case with heavy people, especially those approaching middle age. Superfluous fat is unattractive on any part of the body, but a protruding belly is not only very unsightly but also a great health hazard. This extra fatty tissue puts an added strain on the heart and interferes with the healthy functioning of the other organs. A flat belly is a sign of health and youthfulness.

Yoga exercises tighten the abdominal muscles as the fat breaks down and melts away—something which weight loss in itself cannot achieve. The Locust, Bow, and Abdominal Lift, plus slowly raising and lowering both legs in a lying down position, such as the Shoulderstand, are especially effective for firming the abdominal muscles.

Too often, overweight people become discouraged because their excess weight is an obstacle to performing the exercises. They come up with all kinds of excuses why they have to discontinue the course, or they promise, "I'll return if I lose 20 or 50 pounds." I listen to their rationalizations, their promises of good intentions, but I know I will never see them again. Too bad, because they don't give themselves a chance. Marian was one of the exceptions. She was a woman in her forties, with a pretty face but the proportions of a hippopotamus. A rough estimate would put her weight somewhere around 250 pounds. My heart sank as I watched her attempt the exercises with much huffing, puffing, and perspiring. Fearing the strain on her heart, I could only caution her not to overdo it. She never missed a single lesson. After the course was finished, she reenrolled in the ensuing courses. She still huffed, puffed, and sweated profusely, but her agility had increased to such an extent that she was able to perform the most advanced postures as well as the skinny girls could. It was amazing to watch her, because she defied all the laws of probability. She had gained agility and firm muscle tone but, as far as I could tell, had lost no weight.

During my classes, I discuss various pertinent subjects, among them proper nutrition and weight control, but Marian and I never discussed the subject between ourselves. I'm always available to students who wish to talk over something private with me, but Marian never approached me about losing weight. Often tempted to bring it up, I never did, because I knew there was no sense suggesting she lose weight when she wasn't ready to. Incentive for self-improvement must come from within—it can't be imposed from without. Often the sense of accomplishment that comes from practicing Yoga sparks the desire for still further achievement, as it did with Marian.

After practicing Hatha and Raja Yoga eight months in my course, she moved away. Once she wrote me that she was continuing to exercise on her own. Not too long after that I had a visitor in my class who looked familiar but whom I couldn't quite place. It was Marian back on a visit. She looked marvelous. The reason I hadn't recognized her was that she had lost 100 pounds. By patiently continuing Yoga, but not driving herself, she gradually and naturally had found the incentive to lose weight. To help her along, she'd joined a dieting group.

Marian is one person who will keep her excess weight off, because in Yoga she found a substitute for gluttony. How many times have you heard dieters complain, "Taking weight off isn't the problem, it's keeping it off"? Theirs is a nerve-wracking battle with excess weight that's like a Yo-Yo: first it's up, then down, up again, down, and so it goes. When you lose weight in conjunction with Yoga exercises, the struggle is not so discouragingly uphill all the way. As I mentioned, many of the tensions that cause compulsive eating—that constant nibbling, that insatiable appetite for something more—are relieved. In addition, the more you do the Yoga exercises, the more the desire for huge quantities of food and for heavy, fattening food decreases. Your body, beginning to get into shape, doesn't want to be burdened with a lot of heavy food, with the result that your willpower is bolstered immeasurably.

I was quite heavy through childhood and part of adolescence, but by the time I was eighteen I'd become fed up with the boys treating me as their chubby pal. With what seemed heroic self-denial, I managed to lose most of the excess weight in an effort to transform myself into a femme fatale. Fortunately for me, at that time our standards of shapeliness were set by the proportions of Betty Grable rather than skinny fashion models. After that, I never did regain what was kindly referred to as baby fat, but I was always fifteen to twenty pounds above my present weight. Now I am slim but certainly not skinny. As I became more and more serious about Yoga, my weight loss occurred not so much because I wanted to lose weight but because I actually desired less food. I no longer wanted to eat a lot of rich, starchy foods, because they settled uncomfortably heavy in my stomach and interfered with the proper execution of most exercises. It is preferable to start out doing Yoga without the hindrance of extra poundage, but those who begin overweight and stick with Yoga will most assuredly gain the incentive to lose weight. And once they've lost those extra pounds, Yoga will help keep the pounds off.

Well-Proportioned Figure

Those who ask, "Can I lose inches by doing Yoga? Can I develop a more beautiful figure? Can I become better proportioned?" I answer with an emphatic "Yes."

A lot of people start Yoga because they want to get rid of a certain bulge here or there. They ask me to teach them only exercises for that particular area of the body. What they have in mind is spot reducing. Judging from the ads usually found in the women's magazines, the market is filled with slenderizing salons to achieve miraculous spot reducing. I had firsthand experience with the effectiveness of an electrical massage machine at a health club once when I was trying to reduce unsightly fat on my outer thighs. After three months of religious devotion to that machine I had worked off the bulge. It had disappeared from my thighs completely—only it had settled higher, increasing the dimensions of my already opulent hips. Which left me only to chalk up another plus for common sense. Instant gimmicks are no substitute for overall effort.

There are Yoga exercises that direct attention to certain parts of the body, such as the Arm Roll for the upper arms, the Standing Twist for the waist, and the Pelvic Stretch for the hips. However, effective spot reducing—and when I say effective, I mean that the bulge is gone from your body, not merely pushed somewhere else—is accomplished by working the entire body and not excluding any area, even those areas you happen to be proud of. With overall Yoga exercises you get the special bonus of not only eliminating a specific ugly bulge but of streamlining the entire body. Provide your body with proper exercise, and it will rehabilitate itself. It will set to work intelligently to achieve its proper proportions. It will know where to subtract superfluous inches and where to add required inches.

Yoga can't accomplish miracles. It can't make a tall person

short, for instance. But, with intensive stretching, it can make a short person a little taller, as was joyfully reported to me by Irene, one of my students, who grew from five feet to five feet one inch after a year of Yoga. Irene had not particularly concentrated on adding to her height, but in the process of doing all the exercises she had added an inch.

Most people aren't so much concerned with adding inches lengthwise or widthwise as they are with subtracting them or pushing them around to end up with the right proportions. I used to be the classic example of the out-of-proportion figure, with the most generous share of bulk in my hips, buttocks, and thighs. Anyone similarly proportioned knows what a hard time I had finding clothes to fit me. And once I did find something to fit me, the way I looked in it was nothing to brag about. I wore slacks only when absolutely necessary, and skirts didn't look much better on me. Before starting Yoga I wore a size 14 top and size 16 bottom. After graduating to a size 12 top and 14 bottom, I finally achieved the status of a perfect size 8, including skirts and slacks. After my initial weight loss, I did not lose another pound. I weigh 120 pounds and am five feet four inches, yet I am considered petite—quite a change from someone who used to be referred to as "that big girl."

Yoga enables the body to mold its basic structure with an innate loveliness.

Firm Muscle Tone

An attractive body is a firm one. "Young" and "firm" are words that inevitably go together, just as "old" and "flabby" do. Firm muscle tone, without unattractive bulging muscles, is achieved by Yoga's method of stretching the muscles, holding them motionless, and slowly releasing them. Muscles are there to be used. The more they're used the better shape they're in. But when less and less demand is made on our muscles, as is the case today, when people's activities consist mainly of riding, sitting, and turning dials, the muscles deteriorate. They lose their resiliency and get flabby. And let me say a word to the housewife who's indignant because she's probably reading this after spending the entire day on her feet, cleaning, cooking, ironing, and getting what she considers plenty of exercise. Maybe no one can accuse you of inactivity, but that doesn't mean your muscles are getting the proper exercise. In housework very often muscles receive the wrong kind of exercise and many muscles are neglected altogether. The same applies to a great deal of physical labor done by men. Yoga provides beneficial exercises aimed at all muscle groups, even those rarely used. Some exercises are overall firmers, such as the Head Knee Bend and the Complete Leg Stretch. Others concentrate on neglected areas, such as the Arm Roll for correcting flabby upper arms and the Side Stretch for firming muscles on the sides of the body. Remember, it's always easier to keep a machine in good condition than it is to repair it after it's been damaged. And that especially applies to the human body.

If you've been carrying out a steady program of swimming, for example, you're probably in good shape. You'll enjoy doing the Yoga exercises to keep firm. But if your muscles are losing their elasticity, causing your body to age much sooner than it should, right now is when you should counter the effects of time through Yoga. I'm not promising that Yoga will make a forty-five-year-old woman look like an eighteen-year-old girl, but it will certainly promote a youthful face and figure.

Often people who consider themselves overweight appear much slimmer once their bodies have firmed up, eliminating the necessity to lose large amounts of weight. And if you are dieting, Yoga exercises help keep the skin from sagging while the pounds drop off.

Whatever your age, Yoga can keep your body in its best condition.

Healthy Skin

Women spend millions of dollars annually on creams and lotions that promise them beautiful, radiant complexions. They could save themselves a lot of money, time, and disappointment if they would only realize that what goes on top of their skin is less important than what is going on beneath it. The most effective cosmetic for a glowing, healthy-looking complexion is good circulation, enriching the tissues of the skin and eliminating toxins that cause skin eruptions. Many of the Yoga positions practiced in conjunction with proper breathing are designed to do just that by stimulating circulation and purifying the blood. Especially effective are the inverted positions, such as the Headstand, Head Knee Bend, and Shoulderstand, and all the breathing techniques.

Erica, who had pretty features but a sallow, dull complexion no makeup could hide, is a good example of the effects of Yoga on the skin. It was only a short time after she had started Yoga lessons that she told me, very pleased with herself, "People have been telling me how well I've been looking lately." I wasn't surprised. The change was obvious to anyone who looked at her face, for Erica's once unattractive complexion now had a beautifully healthy glow.

Physical well-being is the world's greatest cosmetic. I'm not forgetting good diet, which is essential for healthy skin, but I'll get to that in another chapter.

Good Posture

Did you ever admire a beautiful girl sitting down and then watch her get up and shuffle away, hunching her back and dangling her arms? Didn't her physical beauty and appeal slip away with every step she took? Or did you ever observe someone who sat, stood, and walked erectly and gracefully, who did not really possess extraordinary beauty or an ideal figure but was able to create an impression of both through perfect posture? Think of an older person you know who looks younger than his age. Isn't it his straight back that makes the difference? Not only does he look younger, he most likely feels younger, acts younger, and is healthier than his stooped contemporary. Yes, good posture goes hand in hand with beauty and youthfulness. And the key to good posture is a strong, healthy spine, one of the prime objectives of Yoga exercises.

As man evolved from a creature that supported its weight on all fours to one that walked upright, his spine did not strengthen sufficiently to always bear comfortably the burden of the upright body. That is probably why we are so prone to backaches. Women especially suffer from backaches and spinal maladies, because of the additional strain that results from carrying their babies in a vertical position during pregnancies and carrying them in their arms after birth. We do seem at last to be learning from primitive tribeswomen that carrying a baby on the back helps prevent spinal disorders and sagging abdominal muscles. More and more smart mothers are using the devices on the market that facilitate transporting the baby papoose-style.

I've observed that more attention is paid to developing healthy spines in the young in most European countries than in America. German schoolchildren, for instance, as well as children in other parts of Europe, carry their school books in a satchel on their back, use a knapsack to carry anything heavy, and are required in school to do exercises to strengthen their back muscles. In this country the commendable habit of carrying school books on the back seems to have vanished with the bustle. Pictures of bygone days show children walking to school with their book straps slung over their shoulders, in contrast to today's children who hunch over heavy books carried in their arms. I hope that one of these days parents and educators will take measures to correct this seemingly innocuous habit, which I have no doubt is impairing the posture and general health of our children.

My father had the German fervor for good posture. He was quite short, but by constantly holding himself erect, he gave an illusion of height. He had a favorite saying that contains much truth, "One cannot think straight unless one walks straight." Unfortunately, he carried his passion for good posture to the point of obsession, incessantly nagging me to stand straight. As so often happens, his constant haranguing produced exactly the opposite effect. To defy him, I turned into a slump. It seems that all my life there was some well-meaning soul who slapped me on the back and told me to straighten up—and whom I could have cheerfully killed. My already poor posture became even worse with my back injury, aggravating and slowing down the healing process.

But where everything else had failed, Yoga succeeded. First of all, all the sitting and standing exercises begin with the head, neck, and spine in a straight line. This is useful to remember any time you want to check on your posture. By straight line, I don't mean as rigid as the guards at Buckingham Palace. Keep straight but relaxed. The person who tries to maintain good posture by keeping his shoulders and spine constantly stiff is putting added strain on his back. Secondly, many Yoga exercises concentrate on strengthening the spine—for example, the Alternate Leg Stretch, the Plough and Twist, the Dancer's Pose, and the Shoulderstand. The stronger your spine is, the easier it is to maintain good posture. The third way Yoga helps with posture is a subtle one. Yoga makes great use of the imagination. As you're doing the exercises, you're expected to think of yourself as beautiful, moving with grace, standing tall. I'd say it's nearly impossible to think of yourself in those terms and still slouch.

Gradually, good posture has become a natural habit with

me, as I have seen it become with many of my students. I wish I could tell you that after forty years of slouching I've completely transformed myself and stand, sit, and walk straight at all times. But to be perfectly honest, once in a while I do catch myself reverting to sloppy posture, because it takes time to undo a habit the body has spent decades establishing. However, correction is a simple matter of reminding myself, and then I'm straight again. Most people's poor posture is a habit. Once Yoga has enabled the body to establish the habit of good posture, you'll find it much easier to rid yourself of the habit of bad posture.

Flexibility

A flexible body is a young body. The Yogi knows that he can slow down the effects of time on his body by emphasizing exercises that maintain flexibility. An old body moves stiffly, a young one with fluidity and ease. The difference between the two lies primarily in the flexibility of the spine and joints. Men in general are much less flexible than women, even if they are young, athletic men—sometimes *because* they are athletic. Athletic men often put too much emphasis on developing only certain parts of the body, especially the muscles in the arms and shoulders, while allowing other areas to become stiff with age.

Because flexibility is so dependent upon the elasticity of the spine, Yoga concentrates on gradually stretching the spine in all directions with a variety of positions. Exercises like the Standing and Sitting Twists give the spine a *corkscrew* kind of workout. The Alternate Leg Stretch and the Plough, for instance, stretch it forward, the Bow and the Camel backward. Notice I said *gradually*. The first few times you do an exercise like the Alternate Leg Stretch you'll probably think your spine isn't responding at all. It is, but little by little. Each time you work out your spine, it gives, and regains more youthful elasticity. The degree of spinal stiffness is an indication of how badly it needed the exercise. Fortunately, the spine is constructed in such an ingenious fashion, with each vertebra hinged to the next, that it can become resilient once again regardless of its age and rigidity. But continuous systematic exercise is essential.

In addition to spinal flexibility, Yoga emphasizes flexibility of the legs. Probably the position that comes to most people's minds when they think of Yoga is the familiar cross-legged Lotus Seat, so effective for loosening up rigid leg muscles. It's been my observation that the leg muscles are stiffer than the spine and take more time to limber up. The most rigid joints in the adult body tend to be those in the knees, where mineral deposits tend to build up. Exercising the knee joints breaks down these deposits, allowing the blood to flow through the area naturally. The stiffest tendons seem to be the hamstrings, at the back of the knees, as you will soon learn at your first attempts to exercise them. Don't be discouraged; the initial discomfort is natural and will soon pass.

I have found that the time spent in achieving the Lotus depends on an individual's bone and body structure. Some students who may be stiff otherwise can attain the Lotus position easily in a short time. However, the majority have to put great effort, usually accompanied by much creaking and groaning, into the preliminary exercises such as the Leg Bounce and the Thigh Stretch that I teach to limber up the legs. I am most sympathetic but optimistically persistent, for if I, who owned the stiffest pair of knees to ever attempt the Lotus Seat, could achieve it, so can anyone. Time limits should be forgotten. Remember you're receiving benefits from working toward the position even before you've actually achieved it. It may take as much as a year to attain total flexibility of the legs, but you'll find it well worth the effort. Not only does the Lotus put new bounce in your legs, but it shapes them into lovelier contours.

With every passing day the Yoga positions, which at first looked like impossible acrobatics, become easier. When the first suggestion of resiliency inevitably appears, there comes the feeling that what seemed hopeless to achieve at the start is, after all, possible. To those with patience and persistence go the rewards of Yoga. Flexibility cannot be obtained overnight, once it's been lost, but everyone, regardless of age, sex, or the stiffness of his body, can become as supple as a child.

Grace

The most eloquent evidence that Yoga leads to grace is the fact that many of my students ask whether I used to be a professional dancer. I am very flattered, but I must answer truthfully, and without false modesty, "I used to be a professional klutz."

In a photograph taken of me at age seven, in ballet school, I am completely hidden by the other children, except for my face sticking out, because the ballet instructor was ashamed to show me. With good reason: I looked like a baby elephant in a tutu. And I danced like one. In school gymnastics, which were taken most seriously in Germany, I was an utter disgrace, because of my clumsiness. As an adolescent, I never pursued any of the sports my parents had forced me to learn—swimming, bicycling, ice skating, tennis—because of the way I looked performing them. With time, I lost some of these adolescent inhibitions. While not exactly cutting a sporting figure on the skating rink or tennis court, I learned to laugh at myself. Not very heartily, I admit, but gamely. I had resigned myself to gracelessness. Yoga, however, operates on the assumption that the body is meant to move with grace. This applies not only to women but equally to men. Rather than detracting from manliness, grace adds to it. The exercises are a series of graceful movements, gracefully executed. Again, your imagination is called into play. As you perform the exercises, think of your motions as flowing gracefully. This ease of movement will indeed become a reality as your body loses its stiffness. Exercises like the Dancer's Pose and the Basic Stretch train your body for grace. You'll notice how these and other Yoga positions resemble dance movements. Actually, every Yoga position can be made into a dance movement, and every dance movement can become a Yoga position. No doubt this is why those of my students who have had previous training as dancers can naturally execute most Yoga positions. However, it isn't necessary to be a dancer, for even those who walk into Yoga with two left feet can learn to move beautifully.

Poise

Poise is grace plus self-assurance. In Yoga we sit, stand, and move with poise until it becomes part of us. The physical poise of the body eventually results in dignity and ease of manner in dealing with people. It is easily recognized and appreciated by others, because those who possess it radiate an aura of calmness, favorably affecting whomever they come in contact with. The slow, sometimes almost languid movements in Yoga, combined with the stretchings and balancing of such positions as Simple Fish, Dancer's Pose, Shoulderstand, and Headstand, all foster poise. In addition, the confidence we gain as we attain the more difficult poses leads to more poise.

Coordination

It is taken for granted that coordination makes the difference between mediocrity and excellence in any sport. However, good coordination is a factor that affects how well and efficiently we perform any physical task, including driving a car, playing the piano, or wallpapering the bathroom. Most people believe that, like freckles, you either have it or you don't, and there's not much you can do about it. The Yogi doesn't take such a negative view of coordination, or for that matter, any physical attribute. The body was designed by nature for good coordination; therefore, if the body is lacking this quality, Yoga will lead the body back to coordination.

When I jumped out of the window during the fire, I landed feet first. I am positive that had I had Yoga training at that time I would have been able to guide my fall to minimize my injuries. I had always had poor coordination, yet today I can execute some of the most difficult Yoga positions, including those bordering on acrobatics. Not only can I get into them, but I am able to remain motionless in them for some time. (See illustrations at the end of the book.) I cannot think of any Yoga exercise that does not produce coordination, the most effective being the balancing exercises such as the Dancer's Pose, the Basic Stretch, and the Headstand.

Symmetry

Yoga also helps restore physical symmetry. It may come as a surprise to some people to learn that their bodies are uneven. For instance, if you have ever gone to a chiropractor you may have been greatly alarmed to hear that one of your legs was shorter than the other or one shoulder higher than the other. If so, you're not unique, because everyone's right and left sides are different. The chiropractor attempts to restore symmetry through manipulation. So does Yoga. During the Yoga exercises these imbalances become especially evident, because everyone discovers it is more difficult to assume and maintain the positions on one particular side than on the other. By exercising the entire body, we can concentrate on the side that needs most attention, correcting the imbalance.

Pleasing Voice

Often a person is summed up in the description: "She was pretty until she opened her mouth to talk." A pleasant speaking voice influences more than we realize the impression we make on others. People who knew me before I started Yoga tell me that the quality of my speaking voice has changed, that it has become softer and more melodious. I attribute this to the stimulation of the vocal chords by the Complete Breath, Bellows Breathing, and the other breathing exercises. In the past I had never submitted my fellow man to my singing. Now, although I doubt that I ever will be competition for Joan Sutherland, I can try Yogic chants before my class without causing my students pain.

Vitality

The most attractive people we know are vibrant and alive. They're ready to tackle anything, can accomplish more in a day than some people can in a week, enjoy life to its fullest and glow with what seems to be a never-diminishing supply of energy. Unfortunately, too many people never have enough energy and don't know how to increase their supply.

Physical energy is usually equated with strength, which in turn is confused with bulging muscles and the ability to lift great weights. But intensive muscle development and weight lifting don't serve too much purpose in everyday life except to a boxer or a weight lifter. What, then, is energy? Energy is power. Put in human terms, energy is the power that enables the body to function at a high capacity without undue fatigue. Really, energy should be equated with staying power or stamina.

In Yoga we strive for a body strong in stamina. In the same way that we can release energy through chemical changes, we can produce energy in the body through physical change. Yoga, more than any other form of exercise, can produce this energy most efficiently and with the least amount of strain to the individual. Everyone has potential energy stored within his body which does not release itself but requires definite effort to set it to work. Yoga stretchings, manipulations, and breathing release this untapped energy, thereby vastly increasing one's endurance and vigor. We are thus provided with a steady stream of energy that carries over into our work and all other activities.

I realize it sounds incongruous to the Westerner that the slow, gentle movements of Yoga can increase vitality. We've been brought up with the misconception that any exercise that doesn't exhaust you isn't doing you any good. I am of the opinion that any exercise or sport which produces excessive strain or fatigue is not only ineffective but harmful. The Yogi believes in conserving energy. It just doesn't make sense to expend huge amounts of energy in order to gain energy. Yoga exercises are designed to enable the body to produce more energy while retaining the supply it already has. In this way the body is fortified with reserves of energy, available when needed.

Let me differentiate between the steady, flowing quality of Yoga energy and the sporadic bursts of so-called nervous energy. Caffeine, alcohol, and sugar may all give you a quick lift, artificially stimulating the body for a short time. But the energy gained from these sources wears off soon, often leaving undesirable side effects. The same is true, to an even greater extent, with "pep pills," which leave a person feeling even more tired after the stimulation wears off. So he swallows another one, feels supercharged for the six, eight, or ten hours the drug is effective, and then experiences the inevitable letdown. Gradually, he becomes dependent on the pill for his energy and feels he cannot function without it. In differing degrees, these artificial stimulants are all jarring to the system, and the system reacts with increased tension, insomnia, and often serious malfunctions. Also, these people who are in a perpetual state of being "souped-up" may talk and move a lot, producing much sound and fury, but they usually accomplish much less than the people who quietly move through life with an even flow of energy.

Most of us are aware of how tension drains our energy. Again, attacking tension with tranquilizers only produces a temporary artificial effect without solving the problem. Stretching and breathing away your tension with Yoga releases the energy that has been pent up and immobilized by stress. With less tension we're better able to handle the annoyances and frustrations that beset all of us in our work and our relationships with others. By using less energy to cope with these situations, we're conserving more energy for our storehouse of vitality.

The body can be quickly refortified with Yoga in much the same way a battery is recharged. In cases of tiredness and mental fatigue after a hard day's work, ten minutes of Yoga can act as a complete revitalizer. Particularly effective are the Bellows Breath, Complete Breath, Abdominal Breath, Basic Stretch, Shoulderstand, Cobra, and Headstand. Anyone who learns to stretch out on the floor in the Complete Relaxation, instead of flopping on a bed or couch when tired, will experience an immediate return of energy. Yoga exercises stimulate us to greater capacities for physical and mental achievement. We perform better for longer periods of the day without getting tired, adding years to our active life.

Sleep

It stands to reason that no one can be bursting with vitality without adequate sleep. And all too often it's hardest to get a good night's sleep when you need it most. There are even times when the quality of a person's sleep is so poor that even after sleeping for hours, he wakes up feeling as tired as he did when he got into bed. This is because the body and mind are still keyed up from the day's activities. You haven't given them a chance to unwind. You may not even know how to go about doing that. Inexplicable but true is the fact that the same exercises and methods of relaxation that provide extra energy also promote sound sleep by "unwinding" your body and mind. Practicing the Cobra and Pranayama before bedtime are especially conducive to sleep. When you improve the quality of your sleep you actually require less, because the sleep you do get is completely restful.

One of the modern health myths of our society is that adults require eight hours of sleep. Some people do need that much or more, but for many people six hours or even less of deep sleep is completely adequate. I always used to be tired, no matter how much I slept. Waking up tired, I would drag myself around until my afternoon nap. At night I couldn't fall asleep. In the morning I couldn't wake up—a vicious circle which was aggravated by barbiturates. One of the benefits evident to me after only a short time of serious Yoga practice was the ability to fall asleep immediately, wake completely rested, and function longer on less sleep. Any poor sleeper who practices Yoga will find himself freed from the debilitating cycle of not being able to fall asleep at night, waking up tired, being too tired and tense to fall asleep in the evening, waking up still more tired, and so on to exhaustion. Yoga will make it possible for you to fall asleep with no trouble and wake thoroughly refreshed.

The benefits I've listed are not added separately like beads on a string, each one separate from the other. Rather, the effects of Yoga are cumulative. Take flexibility, for instance. As you gain flexibility, your posture improves; at the same time so does your grace, poise, balance, and coordination.

No magic genie is going to pop out and bestow these benefits on you. You'll have to work for them, but once you get started, you'll want to continue. Your own body will insist that you keep at it. Consistency will pay off. You'll reap the benefits of your diligence with dividends in beauty.

5

YOGA
AND
INDIA

THE EXOTIC EAST has always fascinated Westerners as a land of mysterious cults and the fount of ancient wisdom. If the answer to life were to be found in any geographic location, surely it would be in the remote peaks of the Himalayas. Those who have gone to India have been both attracted and repelled by that vast land. They have admired its lavish palaces, its remarkable diversity, the graceful sari-clad women, and the most beautiful building ever constructed to memorialize a man's love for a woman, the Taj Mahal. They have also been appalled at India's backwardness, poverty, filth, and apparent callousness toward the teeming masses who are born, live out their whole lives, and die on the streets. Through the centuries this interest in India has not subsided.

Today this fascination seems to have reached a peak not only in the United States, but in England, France, and much of Western Europe.

The influence of Eastern thought on American action was so widespread in the sixties that Guruism or Guru worship became the new religion of the seventies. Young Americans dressed themselves as Sikhs in white robes and turbans or in saffron saris and other garb. They let their hair grow long or shaved it off completely. Children born John and Mary or Bob and Nancy were renamed Gopala and Devi or Rama Das and Satya, after legendary Hindu gods. Young people proclaimed their love for an Indian-born teacher and his god, or for the teacher as God himself.

For many, especially the young, Yoga became synonymous with Indian or Hindu cultism. In most Yoga associations in the United States which have been founded or headed by Indian Gurus, Sanskrit prayers and chants and Hindu rites take precedence over Yoga exercises and breathing techniques. Guru worship and adoration is often carried to extremes. For instance, disciples walk ten paces behind the Master, eat the leftovers from his plate, anoint his feet and perform the most menial tasks to please him. I know several Swamis who persuade their devoted disciples to enter Swamihood, which generally demands celibacy and the surrender of all material possessions to the particular Yoga society. Most demand full allegiance from their disciples, proclaiming that they are the only true saviors of society.

Out of all this confusion of fact and fiction, sincerity and charlatanry, has emerged the legend that India is the land where one finds peace and spiritual fulfillment. Like the hero of Hermann Hesse's *Siddhartha*, written for an earlier generation engulfed by materialism, today's youth long to go to the sacred river and free their souls from bondage. They have been led to believe that the practitioner of Yoga can achieve true self-realization nowhere but in India. The detractors of Yoga also point to India. Their argument goes something like this: If Yoga is so wonderful, why is India in such a miserable condition? Yoga stresses peace, yet India is known for its wild eruptions of violence. Yoga emphasizes the spiritual, but the old maharajahs and nabobs amassed material riches with a cupidity that puts our robber barons to shame. The body should be cared for and properly nourished according to the teachings of Yoga, but the Indian masses are sickly and un-dernourished, with an average life expectancy barely over forty. The very word Yoga means union, but India is still divided by remnants of its caste system and political fac-tionalism. Both the scoffers and the disciples share the delu-sion that Yoga and India are synonymous. It is true that Yoga originated in India, but that was thousands of years ago, when India was in its golden age of culture. Beautiful cities were constructed, many with better sewage systems than modern Indian cities have. A thriving civilization built universities that became centers for literature, philosophy, medicine, and art. Yoga doctrines were an embodiment of the highest knowledge and ethics of the period. But then India fell victim to a series of conquerors, and her ancient glory became merely a memory. Ever since India was granted its independence in 1947, it has been desperately trying to improve itself, but the country is shackled by conditions that have been accumulat-ing for centuries: extreme poverty, a population expanding more rapidly than its food supply, mass illiteracy, and a way of life that in some areas has not progressed for two thousand years.

The only connection Yoga has with present-day India is historical and has no influence on the nation's contemporary life. India's burgeoning masses, struggling to eke out a few cents a day on which to exist, do not live by the precepts of Yoga but by religion, primarily Hinduism. Hinduism forbids the slaughter of cows and other animals, leaving these creatures, often starving and sick, to roam freely through both city and country eating crops, spreading disease, and being a general nuisance. It also perpetuates the caste system, with its degradation of the "untouchables." Although the Indian government has legally granted this group an equal place in society, the ancient restrictions still prevail.

If the way of India's salvation does lie in Yoga, the Indians are not aware of it. There are true Yoga teachers in India, but they are not missionaries spreading the gospel, for the principles of Yoga forbid it. The teachers must wait for the people to come to them. Yoga is not a way of life that can be imposed on anyone; it must be chosen. There is a Yoga saying to the effect that the student who wishes to learn the ways of Yoga will find the teacher. Many legends tell of the Yoga student and Yoga Guru who have never met but at first confrontation immediately recognize that they were meant for each other. From that moment on, the student becomes a devoted disciple of the Guru. In circumstances much less dramatic, each person decides for himself to follow the ways of Yoga. The Indian people are not even in the position of being able to choose.

Yet, the idea that every Indian is a Yoga expert seems to be all-pervading. At one time, when students at the university my daughter Carolyn attended became quite interested in Yoga, the university imported an Indian Yoga teacher. The Yoga teacher turned out to be, in my daughter's words, two "fuddy-duddy, roly-poly" maiden ladies who knew a great deal about Indian cooking but little about Yoga. The university would have kindheartedly kept them as cooks, but it turned out that their papers were not in order, and they had to return to India. There are some excellent bona-fide Indian Yoga teachers in this country, but there are also those hired only on the strength of their nationality rather than their ability.

Those traveling in today's India find little evidence of spirituality. There is worship of individual holy men, especially those who can foretell the future. All over India and in all Indian homes you will find pictures and idols and images of multi-armed and elephant-headed gods, statues, temples and lingams (phallic symbols indicating male superiority) to help the faithful in their worship of Shiva, Krishna, or Rama as the incarnation of God.

Unbelievably complicated religious ceremonies are practiced and there is endless chanting of holy songs, especially at weddings and christenings. These are all traditions, most of them going back to their Vedic beginnings, and the people of India, like those elsewhere in the Orient, are loath to part with tradition.

Indians today are as concerned with materialism as everyone else. While the Western world hungers after spirituality, the Indian middle class is concerned only with acquisitions, and the youth especially are fascinated by everything American, from wristwatches to blue jeans.

Most visitors to India never see a true Yogi. There are Buddhist monks, Hindu Swamis, and those who call themselves Yogis swarming the countryside promising riches, happiness, and fulfillment in the next life in exchange for food and alms. The poorest of the poor generously share their food and possessions with them. There are also the fakirs, performing incredible stunts for money, who are usually confused with Yogis. Anyone who understands the Yogic way of life would never mistake these dirty, disheveled, emaciated men, with their long hair and matted beards, for Yogis. True, the fakir can control his body and perform incredible stunts, such as lying on a bed of nails and walking on glass. He will show you his arm, which he has held up until it has withered. He may even demonstrate how he can be buried for an unbelievable period of time and still emerge alive from his grave.

He does all this for money. Like the carnival sword swallower or geek, the fakir is a professional stunt man and is regarded with repugnance by the true Yogi.

The true spiritual Yogi can perform these same feats, for he has trained his body and mind to master nature, but he never pursues the physical performance as an end in itself. Never would he perform publicly for money or acclaim, for he trains his body only in order to liberate his soul. When I use the term *Yogi* in this book I mean the true spiritual Yogi who believes in and lives by all the rules of Yoga: cleanliness, austerity, non-violence, non-injury, truthfulness, spirituality, and self-knowledge. There are not many such Yogis, but some do still exist in isolated regions, living ascetic lives mostly in the Himalaya Mountains of Tibet and India. These Yogis maintain themselves in fairly primitive conditions, dwelling in stark shelters, bathing in icy rivers, eating the smallest portions of food necessary for their health. They do not descend into the world except on rare occasions, when they feel they have an important message to deliver. Then they come without fanfare.

Otherwise, those sincerely in search of peace and fulfillment must seek them out in their isolated mountain retreats. To become a Yogi under the guidance of these teachers means following rigid rules and discipline for many months. One has to withstand great hardship and practice self-denial that very few can endure, Indians and Westerners alike. You might find it interesting to read the accounts of two Westerners who did submit themselves to the grueling training demanded of the true spiritual Yogi. They were Dr. Theos Bernard, tragically killed in the Himalayas, and Sir Paul Dukes.

India, as well as some other countries, has what are known as Yoga ashrams. These are retreats run on a non-profit, communal basis with the members working together, sharing in the maintenance. These ashrams are found primarily in the Himalayas and are the only places in India where the Yoga practiced is similar to the Yoga in the West. The greatest emphasis is on lengthy meditation and Karma Yoga, but breathing techniques and exercises are included in the curriculum. Different Yoga societies operate ashrams all over the world for the practice of various kinds of Yoga. A businessman, say, who practices Yoga in New York, Oslo, or Paris can find an ashram in his own country where he can spend a few days or a couple of weeks intensively studying Yoga.

From its ancient beginnings in India, Yoga has spread throughout the world. In proportion to the population, there is probably less Yoga practiced in India today than in any other civilized country of the world. The poor masses in India certainly don't practice it, nor is it approved of as a pastime for Indian women. True, Nehru practiced Yoga when he was Prime Minister, but so did Ben-Gurion when he was Prime Minister of Israel.

It is only in recent years that Hatha Yoga has been publicly introduced. A television program focusing on India showed an Indian-born Yoga teacher who lives in London and is quite famous in the West introducing Hatha Yoga to Indians, who wanted to know what it was all about. It is only recently that Indira Gandhi, who is a Yogini, sponsored a Yoga center in New Delhi, making Yoga classes available to the public.

Although Yoga should certainly be acknowledged as part of our heritage from ancient India, it should not be linked with present-day India. Yoga is a modern science, the answer to the needs of contemporary life. It does not belong to one nationality; it belongs to all nationalities alike. My hope is that one day it can be made to serve as one link for world unity.

6

YOGA
AND
MEDITATION

THE PRACTICE OF YOGA can be limited to its physical aspects with very successful results. Many people do exactly this, are completely satisfied, and ask for nothing more. But those who are searching for something else, an inner strength, a philosophy to live by, faith—call it what you will—can discover in meditation the path to spiritual fulfillment.

Meditation is as old as thinking man and is a source of all the religions of the world. From earliest times, religious and philosophical sages have advocated that man set aside a period of time to relax his mind and rest from his mental activities in order to revitalize, reenergize and refresh his body and mind to enable him to cope better with his daily tasks and his environment.

Originally houses or places of worship were built for man to sit in solitude and discover the meaning of life in his innermost depths. As organized religion came about and deities evolved, man shifted his responsibilities from himself to higher powers because it was easier to do so. Houses of worship became a way of identification with individual religions. There still exist churches and temples, pagodas and shrines, and altars and mosques for quiet reflection and meditation. However, in our Judeo-Christian society, churches and synagogues represent separation and inspire the division rather than the unification of mankind.

Meditation became prayer, which means to beg or implore someone or something. In contrast, meditation means to turn within to find the meaning of life in man himself instead of in outside forces. Meditation became reserved for the very few: the saints and sages of history and the monks of all religions, who were free from the distractions of family life and the necessity of earning a living and who could devote their lifetimes to meditation.

There are many spiritual schools of meditation—Zen, Chinese Tibetan and Sufi-Culture, Buddhism and Raja Yoga. They employ different methods and techniques, but the goal is the same; namely, to achieve God-realization or God-consciousness. The apex of meditation is the state of unity with the universe or cosmic consciousness, the state where the body and the ordinary mind are transcended, and the spirit becomes the all. It is the liberation of the soul and the total release from the world of things as they seem. The physical body no longer exists. Body, mind and spirit are one with infinity. In true meditation there is no thought at all. There is only the sensation of utter bliss, joy, peace, and fulfillment. In Raja Yoga the road to meditation is arduous. It requires a spiritual teacher to guide the disciple through the eight roads of preparation: Yama—ethics; Niyama—religious observances; Asanas—postures; Pranayama—breathing exercises; Pratyahara—withdrawal of senses and objects; Dharana—concentration; Dhyana—meditation; and Samadhi—superconsciousness. True meditation has no time limits. Yogis and Zen Buddhists spend hours and hours sitting in meditation. In true meditation there can be no set purpose or aim or goal. There are no boundaries or limitations. There can be no attachment to material desires such as eating and sleeping. There are many stories about Yogic saints and avatars sitting in meditation for as much as four weeks in total oblivion, supposedly acquiring supernatural powers and perceptions. The true Yogi can control his mind to the point where nature has no hold over him and he, in effect, has mastered nature.

For the ordinary mortal this state of meditation is neither feasible nor desirable. Those of us involved in a hectic, competitive society cannot abdicate our responsibilities for a life of meditation. Those who try usually end up in a hopeless dither. However, meditation, without the complexities of Raja Yoga, can provide us with a spiritual oasis and bring peace and perspective to our lives, as I will explain later.

Until recently meditation was remote, mystic, and foreign. Those who professed to meditate were labeled peculiar. At this writing, meditation is very much "in." Everybody seems to be doing it, and some feel left out and bewildered as to what the hullaballoo is all about. Meditation has been advertised, packaged, and sold as a panacea for what ails us and as instant peace and enlightenment available to all, for the proper sum.

I am referring primarily to Transcendental Meditation or TM, the creation of Maharishi Mahesh Yogi. The name "Transcendental Meditation" has been copyrighted, but the fact is that all meditation is transcendental. The ordinary mind is transcended in order to reach a higher degree of mind level. TM is not true meditation. True meditation has only one purpose—identification with the Supreme or God-consciousness. TM is in essence a structured mind relaxation or Mantra concentration and is in no way original, but rather is only one infinitesimal part of Raja Yoga. It is, in the strictest sense, a meditation practice and can lead to higher meditation, but it is very unlikely that cosmic consciousness, which is the promise at the end of the rainbow, can be had for a price.

There are today many pseudo-spiritual organizations and meditation societies. I have counted at least fifty in New York City. Some are profit-making, some are not—but all flourish.

Our youth are constantly criticizing and condemning our present society for its materialism and spiritual poverty. Of course, there can be no arguing with their basic concept that materialism must give way to spirituality if a better world is to be created. In their earnest search for significance, they turn to the mystic, the occult, and extreme Eastern and Western religions, to Gurus and Swamis and meditations. In the seventies we have had more than our share of exotic religions and semireligions. Many of the devotees come to the spiritual experience via the drug experience and merely exchange one extreme for the other. There is no doubt that the spiritual involvement is to be much preferred, because almost all these organizations stress purity and abstinence from drugs, alcohol, and tobacco, and advocate vegetarianism. Unhealthiness lies in the fanaticism that is displayed, which leads away from coping with everyday living and dealing with the reality of the present.

TM has the greatest appeal for white-collar men and women, who can feel spiritually enlightened for a sum without getting involved in cultism or rites, except for the initial ceremony where with Sanskrit prayers they pay homage to the Maharishi's Guru. It has become a fashionable topic to discuss at cocktail parties, and as a cartoon caption puts it, "I will tell you my Mantra if you tell me yours." The procedure is that you bring a flower, a handkerchief, fruit, and $165 for adults, less for students and children, to receive a personal Mantra from a meditation instructor who allegedly tunes in to your psychic vibrations. The Mantra has to be kept a secret and must be repeated for twenty minutes twice a day while you sit quietly on a chair. This is the gist of the matter. All else is reinforcement and lectures, personal check-ups, group talks and TM weekends. To the lay person TM becomes a revelation. The constant repetition of the Mantra *does* produce a meditative state. All the claims of TM can be realized, physically as well as mentally. The blood pressure decreases, the metabolic rate is lowered, the heart rate is slowed down, anxiety and tension decrease. There is better performance and an increase of energy, productivity, skills, intelligence, and general well-being. There is scientific proof by TM physicians, psychologists, and physicists, and a wealth of corroboration in books, pamphlets and television documentaries; there have been scientific experiments on individual meditators with EKGs and other machinery, and testimonials from senators, from stars of movies, the theater and TV, and from sports personalities. In other words, TM works, just as all self-discipline done on a regular basis at regular hours produces favorable effects. When you pay for it and are explicitly instructed on when and how to do it, it is doubly effective. But I am positive that if intensive studies were made and tests taken in other relaxation sequences, the same positive results could be produced.

In all honesty I must say that there is absolutely no harm in TM and that it is mostly a good thing. It has benefited those who probably never in their lives took time out just to sit quietly and do absolutely nothing. It is very effective for extremely tense people, for they find an immediate release from stress. It very often works wonders where tranquilizers and psychiatry have failed. As a structured mind relaxation, it is extremely helpful and can easily be adapted and incorporated into the Western life-style. But to my thinking or anyone else's who has ever been involved in Yoga, it is doubtful whether TM will last. I predict that only those who become teachers will pursue it seriously and that it will go the way of all fads and counter-culture movements. I may be wrong, but I believe that it will either quietly fade away or be superseded by a new mind-blowing gimmick. There are offshoots of TM already in operation, such as "Auto Suggestion" and "Relaxation Response."

For the average American, life is getting more and more difficult to adjust to, and periods of mind relaxation and inwardness are indispensable for everyday coping. TM is successful because it is simple, but it is simple in a meaningless way. There is no depth to it, and there is nothing to build on. It is like a prefabricated house without a foundation. The emphasis is on the mental aspects, while the physical state of the body is ignored. But Yoga is built on a sturdy foundation because the body and mind are a single entity in a continual stage of interaction. TM and other techniques can bring about a temporary change, but Yoga and its application are insurance for a lifetime of mental and physical health.

Meditation should reach the mind via the body, because the body is the more obliging of the two. That does not mean that those who are physically handicapped cannot meditate—far from it; but it is a fact that when the body is in its maximum state of health and is perfectly attuned, meditation becomes much easier. A person with a healthy, strong body voluntarily seeks mental insight. I don't suggest meditation to my students in the first stages of Yoga, but invariably those who reach the intermediate or advanced stage of Hatha Yoga become receptive to the spiritual aspects. When they prepare their bodies, and inadvertently their minds, through the stretching and breathing, they make a natural transition into Raja Yoga. When we reach a meditative state via either Hatha or Raja Yoga, it may not be the true spiritual meditation of the devout Yogi, but it is nevertheless meditation, which can become an integral part of our life structure. Meditation cannot be forced; it has to come about, and it has to be pursued not because "it's good for me even though it's a bore," but because there is a need, a will, and a desire. Meditation or any other self-discipline (on a lifetime basis, not as a one-time fad) works only if it is pleasurable. It may start out as a self-enforced discipline, but to establish it as an everyday routine of our daily lives, we must welcome it and give it preference over other activity, even to the point where we experience a void if we forego it.

True Yoga meditation is neither mysterious nor glamorous. It requires diligence in controlling the mind just as Hatha Yoga does in controlling the body. When stripped of the philosophical and psychological terms that surround it, it is a simple method, as all great truths are basically simple. I can explain it in one sentence: To meditate in Yoga means *to let go of all thoughts.* Contrary to common belief, it is not to contemplate or to speculate but to un-think. This is perhaps the most difficult of all feats to accomplish.

Let me try to explain what is taking place in meditation. Meditation is an altered state of brain activity, and there are many schools of thought about what this altered state really is. Perhaps the easiest way to understand it is to examine the scientifically accepted brain-wave change brought about in biofeedback experiments. Four levels of consciousness have been established; *alpha, beta, delta* and *theta.* Beta is the ordinary waking level of mind, and delta is the sleeping stage. In delta our bodies are at rest, but our mind is not resting at all. The uncontrolled or subconscious mind has taken the reins and is incessantly at work composing dreams. Alpha is the daydream state, a higher mind level than beta, and theta is the highest and most refined level of mind. Beta is the conscious or everyday mind, which is very necessary because we need it to cope with the mechanical and technical problems of day-to-day living. It has access to statistics and can tell us how to handle our business, how much money we have in the bank, what to have for dinner, how to drive a car and so forth. But it is a very limited mind and cannot take care of all our problems. It wants to be working constantly, controlling us at all times. The mind can force someone to think when he wants to stop thinking; the person is a slave to the mind. There are times when thoughts become too much to bear, and oblivion is sought through alcohol or drugs. Often a person will seek a diversion to get his mind off something, and he discovers that he can turn his thoughts elsewhere, but he cannot turn them off. Psychotherapy has taught us that it is most often the quality of thoughts that causes mental illness. The way that we see ourselves in relation to the rest of the world strongly influences our happiness and well-being. Some of a person's thoughts are positive, full of purpose and meaning. Others, very often the greater part, are ineffectual and trivial, dwelling on futile daydreams. Running through the mind are also thoughts of greed, envy, and malice. These do not hurt others if they are kept hidden, but they do harm the individual's own body and mind. These thoughts are like poisons in the system, causing dissatisfaction and sickness. To a degree we can, through Yoga practice of asanas and breathing, learn to control the mind and master it, instead of letting it run free. But when we reach the upper stage through meditation practice, the ordinary mind will have taken a back seat. We will be fully conscious, but the thoughts will have become subdued, less pressing, and more refined. We are resting and relaxing the mind from continuous thoughts; we are able to view them, sort them out, categorize them and channel them in proper directions. We learn to silence the mind and stop its endless chatter, and so get in touch with reality. In the alpha state we gain insight into ourselves and learn to function better and more effectively, and we can be more useful to ourselves and those around us.

Through alpha we progress into theta, the highest meditation, or Samadhi, the superconscious or universal mind. There is complete cessation of all thought, and all Yoga aspirations are fulfilled. It is the supreme union, the merger of body, mind, and spirit into one entity. It is letting go of the apparent self and reaching the true self which is the core of existence. We can cross the boundaries of the gross body which we still accept as the real one in alpha and beta. Through meditation practice we can, as ordinary mortals, experience glimpses of this fourth, and highest, level of mind. It is a very beautiful sensation, a feeling of oneness with the universe, and it can help us to overcome fears and accept our daily existence. But prolonged dwelling in this state is very dangerous for the untrained mind and can lead to emotional breakdown and mental instability.

Alpha is the desired mind level for us to reach in meditation practice, but it should be confined to certain times of the day, because a constant daydream state means copping out and turning off from our everyday duties. Both alpha and theta levels of consciousness and in fact *all* stages of meditation should serve only as reinforcements toward achieving a more meaningful everyday existence.

Through meditation, one can practice controlling the mind until one is the master of the mind. With mastery of the mind comes the power to choose the thoughts that are pleasing and useful. As you work toward this goal of mental mastery, you'll discover that your power of concentration has increased. You will be able to focus your attention more intensely without being distracted, making it easier to accomplish the tasks before you. Each person has within himself the capacity for significant purpose and inner tranquility. These potentials can be realized once the powers of the mind are harnessed into beneficial channels. As thought determines action, there is strength to undertake and carry out what was once considered hopeless. Fears and self-doubts will vanish.

Is meditation in essence a spiritual experience? I believe that it is. I believe that it is the true religion of mankind, which has been overshadowed by organized religion, but which can be rediscovered through the practice of Yoga. I also believe that it is as incongruous to charge money to teach someone to meditate as it is to teach someone to pray. Meditation leads man to the infinite, the union with the divine, whether one calls that God or another name. The divine is sought by searching for the essence of ourselves. By finding ourselves we find the Universal Spirit. The God I speak of is within all of us. He does not single out and reveal himself only to a chosen few, but can be comprehended by all in life who seek him. It is man who chooses God. Through self-realization we discover the highest truth, for God is in man and man is in God. This is in all the holy scriptures written by wise men: "God helps those who help themselves," "God unto thyself," "The kingdom of Heaven is within," and "Thou art That." Many have read these truths but not comprehended them, because they were looking for intricate philosophies instead of simple truths.

All religious scriptures have tried to teach man to seek inward peace through prayer and meditation, but man has deliberately misinterpreted their meanings to shift the blame for his shortcomings onto uncontrollable higher forces. But it is only when man can find the strength within himself without relying on outside forces that a better world can evolve. When he realizes that in himself lies the answer to existence, he can lead a meaningful life. When he stops blaming his failures on Providence and learns to honestly evaluate his faults, he can liberate himself from fear and restore his faith in himself.

All the true prophets and saints were Yogis. They were divine not because God chose them but because they sought and discovered God. Everyone can become a Yogi by practicing inner reflection and meditation. Not all are meant to lead the world, but everyone can become strong enough to lead himself through life with purpose and joy, and, when the times comes, to death with acceptance.

Of course, no special house of worship is necessary for meditation. However, communal meditation and chanting can be a beautiful and inspirational experience. The melodic similarity of Hindu, Gregorian, Hebrew, and Muslim chants leads me to believe that they must have been of one origin. Being a social animal, man derives added peace and joy from sharing his inspirational experience with others. Communal meditation and chanting are done in most ashrams. Perhaps someday, as more people become trained in meditation, there will be meditation centers, instead of individual houses of worship, where man can go freely to refresh himself from his daily tasks. This idea of a nonsectarian, spiritual house may sound utopian to most, but attainable to those who firmly believe in the principles of Yoga.

How to Practice Meditation

Successful meditation is not measured by time. Even five minutes of daily practice can bring results. The ascetic Yogi, of course, meditates for many hours, but the everyday Yogi finds one-half hour sufficient for his needs. Like Hatha Yoga, meditation practice is a purely mechanical process of everyday practice. It is the steady routine that produces the benefits.

Meditation can be done anywhere, but it is most effective when performed in beautiful surroundings. If you're lucky enough to have a garden that affords privacy, by all means

meditate there in mild weather. There is nothing more conducive to meditation than the beauties of nature, as anyone
who has ever meditated on a mountaintop or next to a water-
fall will tell you. Wherever and whenever you meditate, make
sure you choose a quiet place and a time that will not be
interrupted. Try to anticipate and deter all possible disturbances. For instance, take the phone off the hook.

Silence adds to the quality of meditation. Living in a society
high in what the experts call noise pollution, most people
have already learned to block out much of the noise around
them from traffic, the neighbor's plumbing or television sets.
However, complete stillness is not a necessity for meditation,
for inner tranquility will eventually compensate for outside
noises. Symbolically, the perfect position for meditation is
the Lotus Pose. This was adopted by the Yogi for meditation
because in this position the legs are locked and the body
becomes completely still, contrary to the Western style of
sitting in a chair, with legs dangling, where we find ourselves
constantly squirming and fidgeting. However, it is the minority who can sit comfortably in the Full Lotus for any length of
time. Sit in a Half Lotus or cross-legged posture, whichever
you find more comfortable, hands resting loosely on the
knees, palms up. Sitting on a small pillow helps, making it
easier to maintain a straight spine, which is imperative to
avoid sleep or a trance-like state.

It is very helpful to relax the body before meditation. Let
your mind concentrate on your head, relaxing the top of the
head and the brain. Direct your eyelids to become very heavy
as they fall over the eyes. Relax all your features, relax the
neck, release all the tension at the back of the neck. Relax the
shoulders, relax the arms and the hands, relax the torso,
especially the muscles of the back and the vertebrae. Deeply
relax the abdominal muscles. It is very important that there is
no tension or strain in the abdomen. Relax the pelvis, the legs
and the feet.

Meditation is more effective when preceded by Pranayama, which, literally translated, means the control of Prana. Pranayama refers to the various breathing exercises that can aid in quieting the mind for meditation. The body and the mind must be prepared for successful meditation. Harmonious breathing is the most effective way to lay the groundwork.

Although all types of breathing may be used, one of my teachers once told me that the Alternate Nostril Breath is the finest preparation for meditation. Through experience I have come to agree with him and use it exclusively as Pranayama.

In advanced meditation *bandhas,* locks or contractions are also used in Pranayama with the inhalation. The purpose of the bandhas is to lock all the openings of the body to hold the Prana within. This is how it is done. At the start of Pranayama, the eyes and nostrils are closed. The glottis is closed by swallowing, the tongue is curled upward against the upper palate to close off the thorax, and the chin is pressed firmly into the jugular notch. At the same time, the heel is pressed into the perineum to lock the genital openings, and the anal sphincter is contracted. This may sound complicated, but it does come easy with the practice of advanced Hatha Yoga, because contractions are used with many of those asanas.

The steps to meditation are concentration and contemplation. Concentration is fixing the mind on an object or a sound. Contemplation is the next stage, when you can hold the image of that object or sound without allowing your mind to wander. Further, it is the ability to abandon the ordinary mind, or that intangible part of it labeled the ego, and to return deep within yourself, beyond the realm of all thoughts and emotions. You have achieved meditation when your mind becomes a continuous flow devoid of thought. When concentration becomes so intense that that continuous flow is absorbed, when future, past and present become one, and when the essence of knowledge is experienced, that is *Samadhi.*

There are many ways to practice concentration. Perhaps the

easiest way to begin is with object concentration. Gaze at a work of art, such as a picture or a statue, or if outdoors, at a work of nature, a flower, twig, or tree. Any object that is pleasing to the senses will do. Look steadily at the object for about three minutes. Don't let the gaze swerve or outside distractions interfere.

Now close your eyes and transfer your gaze to what the Yogis call the "third eye," the area in the forehead between the eyebrows. Hold the image of the picture as long as you can. Contemplate its color, shape, and substance. The immediate reaction will be quite vivid, but the image will fade and begin to melt away. Try to hold on to it and bring it back. At first this will be difficult, but sheer practice will make this easier to achieve.

When the image can no longer be recalled, let go completely and empty your mind of all thoughts and impressions. After a while you will perceive lights, colors, images, and even metaphysical abstractions. Don't be afraid of them or try to hold them back, but sink into these visions and let yourself float with them.

Don't let any outside thoughts penetrate your meditation. Keep the mental door locked tight to keep away these intruders. They will try to slip in any which way, especially in the beginning, but as you progress in meditation you will become stronger than they and more expert in warding them off.

Concentration on the flame of a candle in dim light or in darkness is also effective. Close your eyes and hold the flicker of the flame in the third eye. Try to steady the flicker. When it recedes, order it back.

I have also found that concentrating on and contemplating your own reflection in the mirror is good training for meditation. Just don't get distracted by wondering whether your present hairdo really is becoming. Regard your image impersonally. Learn to hold the gaze until the picture blurs completely. The mental picture will appear in reverse shades of your actual image, much like a photographic negative. But the outline will be quite definite and easy to hold on to and recall.

Another method of practice for meditation is concentrating on sound—music, the song of a bird, or even a fire siren. One of my favorite meditations is on music (a record or tape), preferably Bach, Haydn or Mozart. After a while, you can develop complete awareness of every note, tremor and nuance. You can learn to listen with every fiber of your body and become one with the sound. In class we practice by humming *Om*, because its vibrations last a long time. Om is the most sacred and profound word in Yoga, said to have been the first sound produced at creation and to be the first sound a baby makes when it learns to speak. It seems likely that the Hebrew *Omen*, which became the Christian *Amen* and the Muslim *Amin*, derived from Om. Hindus use Om as an invocation and also to end their religious services. The Yogi completes his meditation with *Om Shanti* (peace) repeated three times. It is also used as an oral and written greeting and as the closing of a letter.

The word's various interpretations even outnumber its uses. In its Sanskrit origin Om consists of three letters: A, U, and M. They are thought by some to represent the body, soul, and spirit, respectively. Others believe they stand for the states of working, dreaming, and sleeping. Then there are the schools of thought which identify the letters with the three great gods of the one divine being: A for Brahma, the creator; U, Vishnu, the preserver; and M, Shiva, the destroyer.

The word itself, which first appeared in the Upanishads, is also open to a variety of definitions. It can mean the universe, supreme wisdom, the highest achievement, everlasting peace, ultimate fulfillment, or reality. Because there is no single translation, it can have different purposes and meanings, such as God in prayer or a Mantra in meditation. It becomes most effective when used as a Mantra in meditation, repeated over and over silently, or chanted with the accent on the M, or hum. Holding the hum as long as possible creates definite vibrations that the practiced Yogi sometimes hears or feels for hours after subsidence.

We chant Om in rounds, using a low voice and drawing out the last sound. When the sound ebbs away, we concentrate on the third eye. We not only listen to the sound with our ears but let ourselves become enveloped within the sound. By sinking into the center of the sound, we become the sound.

I have discovered that there are almost as many interpretations of Mantra as there are of Yoga. Traditional Yogic writings tell us that only a spiritual master can devise a Mantra for his student and that it is the reward for years of rigorous study and devotion. The Guru is tuned in to the disciple's vibrations, and the Mantra has special psychic powers and must never be revealed. However, in Tibetan meditation, which may be the oldest of all, it is said that Mantras do not act on account of some "magic" nature of their own, but only through the mind that experiences them. They do not possess any power of their own; they are only the means for concentrating existing forces.

Baba Ram Das, né Richard Alpert, a self-proclaimed Eastern Guru, advocates the recitation of "Om Mane Padma Hum" (Hail to the jewel in the lotus flower), and the Edgar Cayce Society uses Bible quotations as Mantras, for example "He Restoreth My Soul." Dr. Herbert Benson, author of *Relaxation Response*, suggests using "One" as a Mantra, and Lawrence Le Shan, author of *How to Meditate,* invented telephone-book Mantras, choosing two syllables at random from two last names and connecting them, as "La-Da." The TM people use seed or sound Mantras which have no meaning: Harum, Kerem, Shaim, to name a few. (Yes, people do tell me their Mantras.) I have, in my Yoga studies, received various Mantras from various Gurus, and I have used them alternately. But a personal Mantra is not necessary to successful meditation; any pleasing word, sound, or sentence can be used.

You may find that concentrating on your heartbeat, pulse, or breath comes easiest for you. Experiment with different methods. Eventually you will find what suits you best. When you start meditation, at first you may feel slightly foolish and self-conscious, even though you are completely alone. You have probably always identified meditation with strictly Oriental practices, quite alien to your own Occidental nature. But remember that you probably had the same emotions about the term Yoga, and now you no longer regard it as some quaint Eastern rite. But meditation, like Hatha Yoga, must be experienced to be fully understood. As you practice, don't be discouraged. Although it is a long road ahead to mastering meditation, you will progress each day along the way. Do not begin with preconceived goals in mind. Meditation is not a planned journey; it is an exploration into the unknown toward the discovery of the true self.

7

YOGA
AND
MENTAL
HEALTH

In Yoga there is no boundary line between mental health and physical health. They are one and the same. The body and the mind are intertwined, the condition of one influencing the other either beneficially or adversely. We are constantly being reminded of the relationship between the mind and the body when our emotions manifest themselves physically. Anger and excitement raise the blood pressure. Fear tenses the muscles and dries the mouth. And every torch singer will tell you how unrequited love makes the heart ache. Conversely, a person with a throbbing toothache will find it difficult to concentrate efficiently on making out his income-tax return. For the brain is only another organ of the body. Its malfunctioning will have an impact on an otherwise healthy body, just as a diseased heart, liver, or kidney will; and vice versa, a physical disorder will take its toll mentally.

Medicine is making headway in letting the mind help solve the problems of the body, but unfortunately it very often goes overboard in holding the mind responsible for a real physical problem that cannot be diagnosed easily. Psychiatry in general still tends to overlook the body as the cause of numerous mental illnesses, despite the mounting scientific evidence that many psychoses have a physiological basis. We are generally aware today that ulcers, colitis, migraines, hypertension, and heart attacks are caused or triggered by mental disturbances. Do we also know how many people suffering from physical dysfunctions such as hypoglycemia, or even more serious illnesses such as diabetes and atherosclerosis, are diagnosed as psychotics or schizophrenics and spend years in psychotherapy or are committed to mental institutions? The major breakthrough in the struggle for mental health can come only when psychiatry and medicine treat the *whole* person, both mind and body, as one unit. As it stands now, both in medicine and psychiatry, the emphasis is on symptomatic treatment instead of complete general, genetic and chemical analysis of the whole person's physical and psychological make-up. Generally, the blame for the overwhelming increase in mental illness is still laid to family structure and environment. While Freudian analysis has taken the back seat, psychiatrists seem to be as successful as ever. Whatever school of thought or whatever therapy is applied at present, individual psychotherapy presents a very limited cure for illness. There are still not enough psychiatrists and psychologists to go around, and they can see only a few patients at a time. Besides being able to benefit few individuals, psychoanalysis is most effective for the physically healthy neurotic, the person who can still function in spite of his problems and, in most cases, do well enough in his work to meet the analyst's fees, which are usually quite steep.

Today more realistic psychotherapy has replaced the schools of traumas and repressions, such as Bioenergetic Analysis, Family Therapy, Psychodrama, Gestalt Therapy, Primal Therapy, etc., which deal with the effect rather than the cause, treating the symptoms of the problem directly rather than considering its origin.

More and more group workshops are developing— unfortunately often devoid of trained leadership—such as Encounter, Sensory Awareness, Transactional Analysis, and Sensitivity Training, to name but a few. If the mental problem is purely behavioral, and, most importantly, if the will to get better is dominant, all techniques can help to an extent. There is, of course, research into other methods of treatment, as for instance the megavitamin theory, said to be very effective in controlling schizophrenia, but the main emphasis and the bulk of the research money are concentrated on developing, producing, and dispensing more and more drugs. They range from sedatives, hypnotics, and antidepressants to psy-chotogenics (used only for severe mental disorders), with tranquilizers in the lead. The latter have become almost a daily staple of the general public, and in spite of present warnings of the dangers in overuse of these powerful drugs, Aldous Huxley's prediction that "we will become a tran-quilized society, no longer aware of political and other dangers" may in time be realized.

Certainly drugs play an important part in controlling mental illness. They have been principally responsible for freeing thousands of people from mental hospitals and making life easier for those who must stay. Drug therapy has replaced brain surgery and electric-shock therapy to a large degree. However, although we are aware of the favorable statistics, we have little information on the physical side effects and dangers caused by many of the drugs: how some of them may produce unexpected reactions, from changes in skin color and loss of hair to damaging deposits in lungs, heart, and kidneys, and even sudden death.

The aims of psychiatry and Yoga are related in their ways of working for the liberation of the individual from forces that inhibit and limit him, so that ultimately man can realize his full potential. As more people become educated about Yoga, its influence will inevitably be felt in psychiatry, and the ancient Yogic theory that mind and body are one entity and must be treated as such will be accepted in mental-health research. While, to the best of my knowledge, Yoga has not yet infiltrated mental hospitals, today a good number of private practitioners have incorporated Yoga techniques as part of their treatment and have found them very successful. I have quite a few students now who have been referred to me by a psychologist or psychiatrist.

So far there is no scientific evidence in this country that Hatha Yoga is an aid or adjunct to treatment of mental illness. However, we have evidence of a two-year study by Dr. Udupu, of the Benares Hindu University in India, who has used Yoga positions and breathing techniques exclusively in overcoming alcoholism and drug addiction in his patients. After six months of Yoga practice, some patients are said to be controlled, arrested, or cured. Formerly classified as strictly physical diseases, both alcoholism and drug addiction have been recognized, to some extent, as mental illnesses, and are generally treated as such, through individual or group therapy and through replacement drugs.

I have also taught and instituted Yoga teaching in drug and alcohol rehabilitation centers. While we cannot reach everyone, we have helped many. Those who accept Yoga have an important tool in rehabilitation and a better chance of staying unhooked when they leave the treatment center. Yoga can teach them to reach within. They can learn to use it as a source of energy and strength whenever cravings or temptations occur. It helps them to integrate the suffering and to become strong and whole again. In all addicts' psychological make-up there is the need for the stimulant in one form or other, and instead of looking for the chemical high, they can substitute the natural high to be found in Yoga. The greatest compliment ever paid to me came from an alcoholic who said to me, after my class in exercise, breathing, and relaxation, "Lady, that was the cheapest high I ever had."

There are practitioners outside the mainstream of orthodox psychiatry who follow the principles of Dr. Edmund Jacobson's progressive relaxation, Dr. Wilhelm Reich's orgonomic psychiatry, or Alexander Lowen's Bioenergetics. These methods involve different theories on mental illness, but basically they adhere to the ancient Yogic wisdom that the mind can be stilled through muscular relaxation. Mental tension corresponds to muscular tension, for all tension originates from a concentrated muscle. Thought, movement, and feeling occur simultaneously. Within the human, thoughts and emotions always produce a muscular reaction. In orgonomy, progressive relaxation, and other similar therapeutic methods, as in Yoga, muscular spasms are either induced by the trained therapist or the patient is taught to induce them himself. Once the subject consciously experiences tension, he can then release it. Tension has become our modern bugaboo. In a less sophisticated time someone would say he had a case of nerves, but now the household word is tension. Did you fail the driving test? Yell at your wife? Come home with a blinding headache? Chances are you'll blame it on tension. For tension has become a dictator, holding its victims in an iron grip. And the more tension is feared, the more it is allowed to get the upper hand.

Yoga teaches you not only how to face tension, but also how to set it to work for you. Through the contractions and holds, the body is tensed, then consciously relaxed, unblocking tensions. You can also learn how to "spot relieve" nervousness and anxiety by practicing the breathing techniques. The fiercest tension can be overcome by quiet and controlled breathing. As tension is chased away, relaxation takes over. These results are achieved by sheer mechanical practice. In contrast to strict Freudian psychiatry, Yoga tries to locate the anxiety in the body instead of in the mind, because it is a much less complex mechanism to work with. Instead of forcing the mind to solve all the riddles of life, we turn to the body because it is much more accommodating and flexible.

Yoga exercises and breathing can do the job of any tranquilizer more effectively, permanently, and harmlessly. I have seen this borne out since I volunteered to teach Yoga to patients at one of our leading mental hospitals. My students are not severely psychotic, but rather voluntarily committed patients, all functioning intelligently and almost exclusively heartbreakingly young. Most of them had been searching for answers in every possible way, but having found no answer, they snapped. They are still searching and are very enthusiastic about Yoga. When a new patient sees me for the first time, the immediate reaction is one of unanimous disappointment at finding a middle-aged lady in leotards instead of a bearded, dhoti-clad Guru teaching the class. But they stay at first out of curiosity, then because they enjoy the classes. They come to me all tied in knots. When I touch them, they are painfully taut, but most are able to respond to instruction. As most of these students can't concentrate very well, I start them off with the simplest basic breathing exercises, which I advise them to practice routinely. In time they loosen up visibly, and their extreme tenseness decreases. But unfortunately very little can be achieved, because while the doctors there tolerate

Yoga, they do not give it support. They put it in the same category as basket weaving—something to keep the patients busy. Some doctors even consider Yoga a form of mysticism and prohibit their patients from attending the classes. Not even caring to investigate the possibilities of Yoga, they offer little besides analysis and drugs. Ironically, these patients are weaned from illegal drugs only to become conditioned to legal drugs.

One well-known psychoanalyst who has long been interested in studying relaxation and breathing exercises as helpful adjuncts to psychotherapy is Dr. Stefan de Schill, Director of Research at the American Mental Health Foundation in New York City, where research on this has been under way for many years. When people are more relaxed, they also become more amenable to psychotherapy, and more progress can be made, he says. Therefore, relaxation exercises, such as certain Yoga techniques, can have a beneficial effect for certain people. For others, pills or tranquilizers are needed to achieve similar results.

Working with Dr. de Schill on this project is Ralph A. Suris, an experienced physical therapist who is quite enthusiastic about the dramatic results he's been achieving with relaxation and breathing. "Letting go is the key," he says. "When a person can learn to let go physically, he's able to let go mentally."

In his treatment of patients with psychophysical problems, Mr. Suris combines Yoga with other techniques, such as Jacobson's method of relaxation. "Most of these patients lack the discipline and self-motivation to use Yoga exclusively," he explains. "Younger patients and those who are more highly motivated respond to Yoga best." Personally involved with Yoga himself, he considers motivation the vital element in its successful achievement. "You can't really get Yoga from anyone. You must live it."

If you went to Mr. Suris to supplement your psychotherapy, this is the kind of treatment you would probably receive: First, you are told to stretch out and assume the position of complete relaxation. Mr. Suris starts with this because anyone who is motivated at all can learn to assume this pose. You remain in the position for five minutes. Then, he begins Jacobson's relaxation techniques to establish the absence of muscle tension. He raises your arm and lets it drop. If he meets no resistance and your arm flops down as soon as he lets go, fine and good. Your arm is completely relaxed. But if your arm remains suspended, he'll point out to you that it's muscle tension "because air isn't keeping that arm up." He might ask you to bend your arm at the elbow to get you to feel the tension in your biceps.

From there, he goes on to the breathing exercises which have a calming effect on the mind. The deep Yoga breathing relaxes the mental condition because of its influence on the nervous system, especially its relation to the vagus nerve. If you have never breathed a Yoga breath, the direct opposite of a Western-style breath, he instructs you how to inhale in three parts—beginning with the abdomen, intercostal area, and neck. After filling up with air to your capacity, you hold the breath to the count of ten, only about two or three seconds, then exhale fully with a little forceful push at the end. As you become proficient in the breathing exercises, you do it in one continuous movement without counting. The breathing exercises are done in a straight-backed chair. Mr. Suris advises his patients to practice them during the working day in a straight chair at the office. Or if the office is large and private, he urges them to lie down on the floor for the Complete Relaxation.

Depending on your flexibility and motivation, Mr. Suris teaches you other exercises. If he considers you a highly nervous individual, he probably doesn't try to teach you the Lotus Position. It's been his experience that his highly nervous patients can't relax in the Lotus Seat, because they are too stiff with tension; but if you're accomplished and have flexible hip sockets, he might have you try the Lotus. What he is striving for in the performance of exercise is a continuous flow of movement. "As I get the patient to relax, he becomes physically and mentally flexible. There's a lot of truth to the saying, 'Action absorbs anxiety.' " The exercises are arranged so you will rhythmically flow from one position to the next.

Although Mr. Suris is convinced that Yoga can be used as an adjunct to psychological therapy, he readily admits that his methods are not generally supported by the psychiatric profession. He believes that there are too many in the profession who are becoming over-reliant on "push-button cures," prescribing pills and giving tests. Yet he has found that there are some doctors open-minded enough to acknowledge the beneficial effects of physical therapy on emotional problems. More often it is the patients themselves who realize how physical techniques have helped them.

One such case was a thirty-year-old patient who was on the verge of becoming a psychotic. He had been institutionalized a few times. Originally he had come to Mr. Suris because of a back problem. Mr. Suris used Yoga exercises with the other therapeutic exercises to treat this man's back, as he does in sixty to seventy percent of the back pains he handles. (He has found Yoga exercises useful for relaxing the back and producing spinal flexibility, particularly the Twist for rotation of the vertebrae in muscle spasms due to misalignment.) This particular patient has progressed so much that he has been able to cut down on tranquilizers and visits to his psychiatrist. Mr. Suris believes that Yoga, with the other relaxation techniques, was instrumental in the marked improvement of this patient's condition.

A large part of Mr. Suris's practice consists of treating back disorders. He knows that organic back pains often cause emotional problems; for instance, a person might no longer be able to function in his job. He even had a case of a young married man who was unable to fulfill his sex role because of back pains. One can readily understand the stresses that such a disability would give rise to. Possibly husband and wife could learn to adjust to the problem via psychology, but by attacking the problem physically, that is, curing the back disorder, the emotional problem is also solved.

Mr. Suris has also put Yoga to work relieving the fatigue of harried businessmen. "When a busy executive is doing the exercises, he's concentrating on breathing and rhythmic motion, not thinking about the half-million-dollar deal at the office. His mind is calm, for while he's physically holding and letting go, he's also holding and letting go mentally. They come to me after a day at the office, a bundle of nerves, with tense, aching muscles. But after a short workout, they say they're so relaxed and refreshed, they could begin another day's work then and there." These people feel not only physically and mentally refreshed, but also spiritually refreshed, Mr. Suris points out. "When you relax the mind and the body, you also give the spirit a life."

Also very much concerned with the spirit, Dr. Joseph H. Gelberman is a practicing psychologist and rabbi who incorporates Yoga into therapy. He is Director of the Mid-Way Counseling Center in New York which, as he describes it, is pioneering a therapeutic approach to mental health, using the principles of religion and psychiatry. Asked why he uses Yoga in the treatment of his patients, he answers simply that it was part of him. "Whatever I am, my profanity or saintliness, hopelessness or hope, wisdom or foolishness, is all brought into my practice. Therapy is not merely a technique. The therapist is not a machine, but a human working with other humans."

Dr. Gelberman began studying Hatha Yoga about thirteen

years ago, because there happened to be a Yoga center next to his synagogue, The Little Synagogue. One day as Dr. Gelberman was coming out of his synagogue, the Swami and his students were also coming out of the Yoga center. Dr. Gelberman invited them all in for a cup of coffee, and they accepted. During that kaffeeklatsch the Rabbi was so impressed with the Swami as a real, unaffected person that the next day he went to him and asked to start lessons. At that time, in spite of three operations, Dr. Gelberman still suffered from varicose veins. He didn't get off to a very auspicious start, because soon after he began practicing Yoga, he fell and hurt himself. Then that summer he experienced a miserable week at a Yoga camp. "It was cold, it rained every day and the food was unbelievably bad," he recalls. "Now the food wouldn't bother me, because when I go to Yoga camp, I fast for three or four days. The body trained in Yoga can get along without food for long periods because of Prana."

Yoga helped Dr. Gelberman's varicose veins and certainly affected his emotional health when he was once more able to painlessly walk, do his work, and move around. "There is certainly a relationship between physical and mental well-being," he said. "Before starting psychological therapy, it is necessary to eliminate the possibility that the symptoms have physical causes. For example, the cause of a headache may be psychological, but it may also be a brain tumor."

Dr. Gelberman uses Hatha Yoga on a patient when he thinks it is necessary and when he feels the patient will respond to it. Sometimes when he sees that a patient is nervous, he will show him Yoga breathing techniques to relax him. Or Dr. Gelberman may recommend that the patient go for Yoga exercises. "However, Yoga is not for the lazy. You must work hard at it and have discipline. It's a daily thing, not something you can try for five months, but something you spend a lifetime on.

"Yoga works because it establishes physical health, which

is the basis for emotional health. The exercises can build up your self-confidence, and naturally you'll feel better. Just as you need a place to live to shelter you from the elements, the soul lives within the body. When the roof leaks, you spend a miserable night.

"However, while physical health is a prerequisite for mental health, that is not to say that you need tip-top physical health to have mental health. I personally feel physical well-being is not enough. The man who's in great physical condition isn't going to find it a help when his wife throws him out, because he can't handle the situation emotionally.

"There are people with physical ailments who can rise above their pains by mental and spiritual strength. To the outsider a person may seem a physical wreck, but his physical problems don't bother him. For example, when Rabbi Akiba was being burned at the stake by the Romans, his disciples asked him why he was smiling. 'Don't you feel pain?' they asked. He answered, 'There may be pain, but I don't feel it, because I am so happy that now I can completely serve God in body, mind and spirit.' " As a more contemporary example, Dr. Gelberman pointed to the late President Kennedy, who was in continuous physical pain but was able to rise above it and conquer it.

"If a person has pneumonia, then has a serious fall, then gets beaten up, then is in an automobile accident, all in one month, he could go insane. But if he has a good attitude, he won't." Dr. Gelberman believes that the mental aspects of Yoga can help people achieve the kind of attitude that enables them to rise above the hardships and tragedies of life. Yoga can enable a person to view his problems objectively and so be better able to cope with them. He feels that Yoga concentration can prevent mental troubles so that a person will never have to resort to psychological therapy. One gains detachment from his self and all his little problems through Yoga.

This Yogic detachment does not signify withdrawal from

society or from personal pleasure, he explains; rather, it is the ability to rise above the petty egocentrism that obstructs effective and creative functioning. "There is a difference between needs and wants. Man has certain needs—food, shelter, sex, etc. He also has certain wants—he wants to live in a penthouse on Park Avenue. Problems arise when the wants are turned into needs. I love this apartment," he said, waving a hand at the warmly furnished room we were sitting in, "live in it, work in it, but if I were deprived of it, I could still go on. I would do my work in a basement. That is the kind of detachment that makes a whole person."

I myself was made "whole" by Yoga, after undergoing analysis. Terrible as physical disability is, the anguish of mental illness is worse. There is no single origin of mental illness, for there are numerous circumstances that can cause it. It can be genetic, psychological, environmental, or arise from stress accumulation. As no one in our society is immune to physical sickness, no one is necessarily exempt from mental sickness. In my case it was evidently the effects of my childhood environment, aggravated by successive shocks to my nervous system all through my life, with the accident and loss of my baby as the *coup de grace*. My symptoms were mostly physical, showing up in dizziness, nausea, blackouts, extreme fatigue, and tremors. After a battery of physical tests proved negative, the cause of my illness was diagnosed as mental, and treatment was advised. As I mentioned, I never wholeheartedly accepted the verdict that my ailments originated in the mind, but continued to insist that their causes were physical. However, I finally did consent to psychotherapy. At that time the crowd of psychiatrists I encountered varied in their methods of treatment by being either couch or chair men. Doctors One, Two, Three, Four, Five, and Six had me assume either a reclining or sitting position, took down my statistics, listened to my symptoms, and dismissed me after two or three sessions because the insurance company wouldn't pay their requested fees. Doctor Number Seven saw me for six weeks for a period of ten minutes each time, prescribing a new tranquilizer for me. When I shyly asked when he would start analysis, he suggested that I really must be crazy if I thought that he would "put you on the couch for the pittance the insurance company pays me."

On to Doctor Number Eight, who had apparently reached a satisfactory financial arrangement with the insurance company. He was a chair man, who practiced the silent method used quite often in therapy then, but fortunately not so much now—he did not talk unless I talked. But I did not talk, because I wasn't allowed to smoke and at that time could not utter a complete sentence without a cigarette in my hand, and because having to sit in a straight chair for fifty minutes caused me considerable back pain. Having recently stopped smoking, he didn't let his patients smoke, lest he get tempted. Instead he chewed gum. So we sat facing each other for a whole year in utter silence—he chewing placidly, thinking, for all I knew, about whether he'd have steak or lamb chops for dinner, and I seeing him as the reembodiment of Hitler, hating him with every fiber of my body. That year I didn't get better, but neither did I get worse. I think my hate kept me going.

Thoroughly fed up with the insurance company, my husband and I found Doctor Number Nine through the clinic of a mental hospital. He let me smoke, was kind, talked to me, and made sense. The day came when I stopped seeing him as my father, lover, friend, and psychiatrist, and accepted him for what he was, a physician. Just as I had learned, as a young woman, to overcome my modesty and appear nude in front of a doctor, I learned to undress my thoughts and expose them. As I removed layer after layer, I found, like Alice in Wonderland, that nothing was as it appeared: black was white, light was dark, the unreal was the real. I learned that nothing is so terrible and frightening when you can squarely face it and learn to evaluate it. I improved, and after two years we parted by mutual agreement.

I was fine if all went well, but when faced with a crisis or difficult decision, my old symptoms would reappear. The dizziness, nausea, blackouts would hit me again, although they were not so pronounced as before. I learned to cope with them just as a diabetic or cardiac patient learns to handle his attacks. In other words, my illness was arrested but not cured. This doesn't mean my psychoanalysis was a failure. In the fictionalized versions of Freudian theory, the heroine in analysis suddenly discovers in an awesome moment of self-revelation that as an adolescent she desired incestuous relations with her father. Once these repressed emotions are brought out into the open, she is perfectly well and lives happily ever after. In real life it doesn't work quite that way. It happens very seldom that a deep-seated neurosis or psychosis is discovered to stem from a single trauma. In general, childhood traumata are falsifications, distortions of infantile fantasies, and are hung on to in order to justify childish behavior. (I was one of the few people who have benefited from Freudian therapy, because my childhood environment coincided to a degree with the social background and way of life upon which Freud based his theory of repression of anxiety and guilt.) Also, finding the cause for the mental suffering does not necessarily effect the cure. Most often, when the anxiety is dispelled, a void is created. Psychoanalysis, in its way, amputates an integral part of the individual, for he has become used to living with his neurosis. A positive substitute is necessary to complete the cure. Yoga provided me with the means to become a whole person again. It can help many others who have completed psychoanalysis and are looking for direction in their lives.

However, Yoga is not limited to mental rehabilitation. Its

greatest service to the cause of mental health can be, as Dr. Gelberman points out, in the form of preventive medicine. People break down as a result of stress. The tragedy that causes one person to jump off the roof merely causes another to make adjustments in his life. Yoga can give a person the strength to make adaptations to life rather than be overcome by its difficulties.

I venture to say that anyone who takes up Yoga in early years will not experience mental illness. Because, first of all, he will be able to keep himself in good physical health. When your physical health is good, you can withstand emotional strain better. How many times have you heard people buffeted about by misfortune remark philosophically, "At least, I've got my health." Good health is a wonderful consolation in times of trouble. It becomes increasingly important in old age. Much of the depression the aged suffer is due to their inability to function well physically. The less they're able to do, the less they try to do, and as a result, their depression becomes more intense. Yoga can help ensure an active old age and is also an exercise an older person can perform, building up his confidence.

Many people go through life wound up tightly, their nerves set to snap at the slightest provocation. Each small strain causes them to lose control; a major strain causes them to break down completely. With Yoga exercises you learn to relax, periodically relieving yourself of the mental tension that inevitably builds up to its overflowing point unless it is otherwise released. Once you have learned the relaxation techniques of Yoga, you can apply them any time they're needed, when you're beset by a crisis or when anxiety threatens to overcome you.

The physical effects of Yoga on mental well-being may seem obvious, but the emotional effects are more subtle. Yoga promotes a sense of detachment from the self that is uniquely

Eastern. While Western thinking stresses the individuality of man, the Eastern mentality views man as one atom in the infinite cycle of life and death. The Easterner does not attribute as much importance to himself as the Westerner does. While the Western aggrandizement of the individual has many advantages, it also places a large burden of responsibility and guilt on him, which he may often find too heavy to bear. Yoga can lift the individual out of this state of constant subjectivity and self-centeredness to a place of detachment where he can view himself and his role in the world with objectivity. He learns to look into himself. He can discover his true self, not the puffed-up image that he often puts forth to others. In searching for the essence of himself, he comes to accept himself for what he is and to have confidence in himself.

Turning within to develop your potential, you can build the emotional strength and independence that enable you to pursue your goals unhampered by petty jealousies, fears, and doubts. To think of something more than your small self can give your life meaning and purpose. Bertrand Russell says, "The man who centers his thoughts and hopes upon something transcending self can find a certain peace amidst the ordinary trouble of life which is impossible to the pure egoist." That is what Yoga teaches and that is the basis of mental health.

8

YOGA
AND
HEALTH

ALTHOUGH THE AMERICAN medical profession is still largely unaware of the therapeutic value of Yoga, Dr. Michael J. Errico, an orthopedic surgeon, and Dr. Warner C. Hall, an obstetrician and gynecologist, are well acquainted with Yoga and were happy to provide me with the following statements.

The human body is a finite structure of amazing complexity, which was designed to last and be effective for approximately fifty to seventy-five years. Like all mechanisms, its component parts are subject to stress and wear, but, unlike many mechanisms, it has a great many built-in self-regenerative and reparative mechanisms and processes. Not all of the chronic wear and tear is reparable, and so the inevitable process of degeneration advances. The most obvious form of this type of wear and tear is seen in the aging of the skin. The full, rich turgor of a child's skin disappears even as adolescence approaches, and as extreme old age is reached, a thinness and flabbiness of the basic skin structure is inevitable. Arthritic changes occur in the fingers. Major joints begin to wear very much as a ball bearing in a machine begins to wear. These are inevitable changes, true, but by good health and care of the body, these changes can be forestalled. These are referred to as the chronic degenerative diseases of old age. They include heart disease, arteriosclerosis, osteoarthritis, osteoporosis, degenerative disc disease, and even such common items as bursitis and tendinitis. A certain tendency toward these chronic degenerative diseases is inherent in the basic protoplasm of the individual organism. In other words, genetic predetermination does play a certain role. This, however, is a minor factor when other causes of chronic degeneration of tissue are taken into account.

Chronic degenerative diseases are advanced substantially by the effects of abuse of the body. The most striking example of this is the effect of smoking on the lungs. Chronic inhalation of these noxious vapors has been implicated as the cause of a large number of degenerative diseases of the internal organs. Smoking has been found to be one of the etiological agents in the occurrence of emphysema, arteriosclerosis, and even bladder cancer. Chronic alcoholism, a major disease of our current society, is well-known for its degenerative effect on the liver and on the brain. Obesity is an extremely important causative factor in the development of arthritis, as well as metabolic diseases, such as diabetes and so forth, which increase these degenerative processes.

It is not as well appreciated, however, that lack of use of the human body can also be implicated in the rapid advancement of these chronic degenerative diseases. Many recent studies on the nature of stress exercising have strongly indicated that cardiovascular function can be markedly improved by use of the body, and that lack of use and subsequent lack of stamina may well be a major causative factor in premature death. The musculoskeletal system is particularly prone to advancement of its degenerative processes by lack of muscular protection and reliance on the passive structures of these joints, such as their ligaments. Firm support of musculature is required as an adjunct to ligamental stability of joints, and one without the other produces a disharmony in the function of joints, leading to early degenerative changes. It is clear to all of us who treat the chronic degenerative diseases of the musculoskeletal system that one of the major causative factors of this condition is lack of proper physical conditioning and of proper exercise.

Finally, the aging process and its subsequent physical breakdown are also greatly dependent upon the mental health of the individual. The Greeks knew that a sound mind in a sound body was the ultimate form of health. Mental strength is the primary foundation upon which physical health is based. Therefore, exercise programs should be directed toward mentally as well as physically desirable effects. In my own practice I have seen the distinct relationship between mental and physical health. Minor or mild physical stresses are frequently perceived as major obstacles which cannot be overcome. A healthy mental attitude can put minor degenerative problems into their proper perspective.

Yoga exercises are particularly well adapted to the relief and the avoidance of chronic degenerative diseases. Yoga is extremely useful in the toning of musculature, the production of resilience in joint structures. Yoga's emphasis on gradual assumption of the physically healthy state is also extremely advantageous to people who have neglected or abused their bodies for long periods of time. Many people who are chronic sufferers of pain from degenerative diseases can gain relief of their symptoms by properly applied exercises. Indeed, many people, such as Ina Marx, who have advanced degenerative changes in their backs or in other structures, have gained complete and total relief for many years by the judicious application of Yoga techniques. The key word here is *gradual*. The second key principle is consistency. As in any exercise, it is incorrect to do that exercise only once in a great while. Persistence allows for the development of a healthy state of body and mind.

Michael J. Errico, M.D.P.C.
Clinical Instructor in Surgery
Cornell University Medical College

For the antepartum obstetrical patient, Yoga has many important benefits, such as helping to control weight gain, improving muscle tone, and preparing for the ensuing labor.

During labor the breathing control and relaxation methods of Yoga are used to produce a more natural type of childbirth, very similar to the Lamaze method popularized recently by many obstetricians.

Postpartum Yoga exercises are most important to get the mother "back into shape." Here the abdominal exercises are most useful to restore tone to the muscles which have been stretched during the pregnancy. I tell my patients to resume Yoga exercises seven to ten days postpartum. Girdles are out; let the muscles work and become firm.

There are also many benefits to be derived from Yoga by the gynecological patient. Yoga exercises are encouraged to reduce the edema often found in the arm following a radical mastectomy.

After abdominal surgery, when the incision is healed, usually seven to ten days postoperatively, Yoga is used to aid the return of tone to the abdominal muscles.

Urinary stress incontinence, a very disturbing disorder for some older women, can frequently be controlled by exercising the vaginal and perineal muscles, thus eliminating the need for vaginal plastic surgery.

Like it or not, the best modern contraceptive available today is the oral contraceptive, the Pill, except perhaps the oral use of the word "No." The most serious side effect is related to thromboembolic disease. Yoga, by increasing the cardiovascular flow through the blood vessels and by preventing weight gain, is a very important instrument in helping to prevent these serious side effects.

Yoga is of benefit to the menopausal patient who suffers depression and cardiovascular changes (hot flushes), thus often eliminating the need of hormone-replacement therapy. The use of the female hormone premarin has just recently been found to lead to a higher incidence of uterine cancer.

The modern woman is more liberated, intelligent, competitive, and aware of her body. The media, via television, billboards, movie ads, etc., bombard the modern female with the image of a trim *Vogue*-type woman. The days of girdles, corsets, and in some cases bras are over. The days of tight pants and bikinis are here. Thus Yoga is becoming even more popular in helping to obtain and maintain this modern female image.

Dr. Warner C. Hall, F.A.C.S., F.A.C.O.G.
Director of Boulevard Hospital
Queens, New York

Medical science is advancing at a rapid rate. There is a vaccination for almost every communicable disease. A submicroscopic virus can be pinpointed and an antibiotic developed to kill it. An organ can be taken from one person and transplanted to save another person's life. Yet with all these dramatic breakthroughs in medicine, the state of health in this country is a sorry one. Our hospitals are filled with sufferers of chronic degenerative diseases such as heart ailments, arthritis, diabetes, hypertension, and asthma. And it's the rare person who, when asked, "How are you and your family?" can truthfully answer, "Fine, thanks." Most people are plagued with a slew of minor-league ailments—colds and other respiratory disorders, allergies, obesity, nervous tension, and digestive complaints. True, people are living longer, but for too many it is an unhealthy old age. Some degree of sickness has come to be taken for granted, while health has become the exception.

Medical science is trying to solve the nation's health problems by developing and prescribing more and more drugs. The right medicine given at the right time to the right person can make the difference between relief and suffering, between life and death. But at the same time, there now goes on an indiscriminate dispersion of powerful drugs that can cause dangerous reactions. Penicillin, for example, was prescribed freely, until doctors became aware of the frightening allergic reactions it caused in some people. Now penicillin is prescribed much more cautiously. Thalidomide was prescribed for pregnant women, until its horrible effects became known. Millions of women take birth-control pills, although they can produce harmful side effects. The pattern seems to be repeating itself with antibiotics. Cases of ill effects from antibiotics are being investigated, and some of these drugs are being ordered off the market. A growing number of scientists are becoming aware that the prevalent overuse of antibiotics and other drugs may be harming not only the individuals who take them, but future generations as well, by possibly affecting the genes.

Common sense dictates that there are times when medicine

is necessary. But medicine itself doesn't cure. All medicine can do is establish certain conditions within the body, enabling the body to cure itself. Every drug is a chemical, and overuse must, of necessity, affect the chemical balance of the body. While a medication may be coping with a situation in one part of the body, it can adversely affect the organism as a whole. Yoga teaches that the solution to the problem of health does not lie in chemicals but in man himself. Man must increase his natural vitality so that his body is conditioned to resist disease. Yet instead of enhancing and relying on the natural powers of his body, man contributes to their deterioration. Blame for his ill health is placed on the atom bomb (an excuse for mental tension), carbon monoxide fumes escaping from car exhausts, or insecticides sprayed on produce. All of these, of course, do contribute to the problem, but they're not totally responsible for everyday ills, aches and pains, and blah feelings. Man, for the most part, creates his own sickness by disregarding nature and abusing his body. The average American shows more concern for his automobile than for his body.

Take a day in the life of a typical New Yorker—I know quite a few like this, and I'm sure you do too. He has a cup of coffee and a cigarette for breakfast, rushes to the office, either gulps down a sandwich for lunch or has an executive lunch consisting mostly of cocktails. In the course of the day he drinks about five more cups of coffee, usually accompanied by doughnuts or Danish. He rushes home, eats an enormous dinner, after which he either sits or lies down to watch TV, and then goes to bed. He commonly suffers from constipation, indigestion, heartburn, headaches, insomnia, ulcers, frayed nerves, or a combination of any or all of these. His medicine cabinet is well stocked with a variety of prescription medicines plus a generous supply of all the three-way fast-acting headache remedies, antihistamines, bromides, alkalizers, tranquilizers, and stimulants. He goes through life swallowing these pills, increasing the dosage as he grows older, to alleviate his sicknesses. In reality he is only aggravating his deteriorating physical condition. He may live a long time like this but will always feel miserable. This is not even taking into account the harm caused by becoming psychologically dependent on drugs. Sociologists and psychologists are pointing out that the inclination of our youth toward drugs is a natural outgrowth of being raised in homes that are increasingly drug-dependent.

The Yogic attitude toward health and medicine is decidedly different. The Yogi considers his healthy body his birthright; he contends that everyone is born with the potential to enjoy perfect health all his life. He does not, however, take health for granted, but cherishes it as a precious gift and devotes part of his life to maintaining it. He does not coddle his body, but neither does he abuse it. As for disease, the Yogi does not follow the extremes of either ignoring its existence or fearing it. He is rarely affected by disease because he has built up the natural resistance of his body. This is done by a healthful diet, exercise, and the mental serenity of Yoga.

Old age is a disease the Yogi tries to ward off. Kept at its maximum peak of good health, the body slows down the process of aging. Not only is the life span extended, but the body and mind retain their youthful qualities for much longer. The death of a Yogi is always referred to in terms of giving up his mortal body because it has accomplished its present purpose. His soul, of course, is immortal and his body its sacred temple. Because the Yogi has devoted thoughtful care to his body, at the time of death it is said to be still the body of a much younger man.

Everybody, of course, is subject to the effects of time, but not at the same rate. At present, medical science knows very little about the process of aging. Our present acceptance of one hundred years as a very old age for a human being may be completely fallacious. There are people in remote regions of Russia and Pakistan who live way past the hundred-year mark because of their way of life, the purity of the air, and healthy nourishment. At age eighty or ninety they look well and are very healthy.

Most true Yogis have a knowledge of the human anatomy and psyche comparable to that of the trained physician. Their understanding is derived not from medical school but from rigid training and self-discipline combined with common sense. Experience has made them completely aware of every part of their inner body—muscles, blood vessels, glands, and organs. They have learned through rigorous practice to isolate and regulate all these elements in their bodies, including those functions, such as the beating of the heart, which are commonly thought beyond the realm of voluntary control.

This last claim used to be met with much skepticism, but experiments with biofeedback during the past two decades have validated these ancient Yoga techniques. Using electronic signals, man can learn to control his heart rate, blood pressure, glandular secretions, and brain waves.

There are Yogis in India and other parts of the world who are known for their powers to heal. Many people turn to them as others turn to physicians. They are scientific men using methods based on the theory that all degenerative conditions are interrelated, that imbalances of the body stem from a common cause. By manipulating the part of the body that is the counterpart of the afflicted part, they work through the body reflexes via the central nervous system. For example, by kneading a nerve in the foot corresponding to one in the lower part of the body, they are able to relieve symptoms in the affected area. Evidently, this provided the basis for what is now termed reflexology, or zone therapy.

While Hatha Yoga as an exercise program is not very prevalent in India, the Yoga postures and breathing exercises as a form of preventative and therapeutic medicine play a part in the health care of the Indian. There are various hospitals and clinics that are using Yoga for healing purposes, and I have met and talked to Swami Gitananda, an American-educated physician and psychiatrist, who operates a large self-contained ashram in southern India. His patients come from all the surrounding villages, and while he also applies standard medical treatment, he mostly dispenses Yoga postures and breathing techniques for various illnesses instead of pills. He claims to be very successful in treating the mentally unbalanced by teaching them proper breathing. He says, "In the States it costs between $100 and $150 per day to treat one patient in a hospital. We have to treat 500 to 1,000 people for that money, and Yoga applied properly can prevent or arrest bad health, most disease and affliction."

Some Yogis are also credited with psychic healing powers. It is claimed that they can effect healing through intense concentration on the diseased part of the body, because they possess spiritual healing powers that can be transferred to the patient. There definitely exist people who have unusual powers—psychic energy, mental telepathy, ESP. One cannot disregard the scientific evidence compiled on Edgar Cayce, who, in a trance state, diagnosed diseases and predicted cures which proved to be valid for strangers miles away. But generally speaking, it seems illogical that any one person has the mental power to cure someone else's disease of physical origin. I believe that people who are healed through laying on of hands, someone's prayers, concentration, or other rites undoubtedly suffer from psychosomatic afflictions. Sickness that is manifested through the power of suggestion can be dispelled through the power of suggestion. It is their faith in the healer and their willingness to get well or their religious faith that effects the cure. Since most diseases are self-induced, faith healing usually works. It definitely, absolutely cannot hurt unless one is devoid of common sense and refuses medical attention when it is indicated.

What I believe is that each person has the ability and the power within himself to invent disease and to cure it, including illnesses of a physical nature.

We all have infinite power within us which we can learn to channel in the right or wrong direction. In Yoga, when you become aware of the flow of Prana through your system, you can utilize this vital energy as an aid in maintaining good health. But Yoga should never be substituted for necessary medical care. It is unlikely that the Yogi who lives in the Himalayas ever needs medical help. If he does get sick, he is self-sufficient. However, the Yogi or Yoga student living in the midst of "civilization" will use his common sense and seek a doctor when one is needed. Or possibly if his condition warrants it, he might go to a chiropractor. In this country the medical profession represented by the American Medical Association has not truly accepted the so-called new professions of chiropractic and naturopathy. In other countries, such as Germany, medical men and practitioners of these other health professions work together, as they should, because both can benefit from their mutual knowledge for the good of mankind. Chiropractic is related to Yoga in that both stress manipulation of the spine to assure perfect health. It can alleviate pain and effect cures in cases of misalignment of the vertebrae, such as whiplash injuries, where orthodox medicine has very little to offer.

The latest deviation from the path of organized medicine is acupuncture. It was at first fought by the A.M.A., but political and public pressure won out; the A.M.A. was overruled and acupuncture was "in." It became demystified and at last surfaced from its underground position. For years and years it had been a hidden, forbidden, mysterious cult, practiced in dingy rooms in Chinatowns. It has now become legalized but confined only to the hands of the M.D. The result has been that American medical doctors, dentists, and psychiatrists have overnight become acupuncturists after a quickie course from Oriental acupuncturists. It has been turned into a "cure" for a staggering list of ailments, from arthritis to ulcers, from ingrown toenails to cancer, from addiction to mental disease, from deafness to blindness. We are not talking about the acupuncture used for anesthesia, which is a different subject altogether. Today the needle is wielded by a significant number of M.D.s, and acupuncture has turned into a lucrative practice. Acupuncture is actually an ancient art of healing which originated in China and has spread through the Orient. The theory is that all illnesses stem from an imbalance of the flow of energy, and that they can be cured or relieved by stimulation of the affected pressure points in the body. This is accomplished by pushing hair-fine needles into the skin and stimulating the needles by various methods, such as twirling or heating. This releases the energy flow, and the body can heal itself. It is an extremely intricate study, originally requiring an entire lifetime, passed on among the Chinese from father to son, from generation to generation. In today's China a three-year study of acupuncture is the minimum requirement. Originally acupuncture was used solely to prevent disease. Every sickness was regarded as a cardinal offense, and the Chinese doctor was paid only when the patient stayed healthy.

Very similar is the Japanese method of fingertip massage, called acupressure or shiatsu, used to activate the pressure points. This is also available in the United States, and those in related fields, such as chiropractors or Swedish masseurs, have jumped on the bandwagon.

Oriental healing methods are flourishing in the United States, and one hears stories of miraculous cures. I don't doubt that they can help in many cases, and I don't think that they can do great damage except in the hands of a complete incompetent, or if dirty needles are applied and cause an infection. But neither acupuncture nor acupressure is a panacea; nothing is—not chiropractic, reflexology, naturopathy (curing disease through proper nutrition), homeopathy (herbal medicine), etc. They all can help to an extent, depending on the patient's confidence in the administrator or belief in the method. Sometimes they help and sometimes they don't help. To get hung up on one method is foolish. It makes sense to have a chiropractor treat a whiplash injury, but it is nonsense to ask him to heal a sore throat. Acupuncture can certainly relieve the symptoms and pain of arthritis, but it can do nothing for an inflamed appendix.

Classic Yoga hygiene includes internal cleansing techniques which are considered essential for achieving and maintaining perfect health. Inner cleansings are thought to be as important as outer cleansings. A devout Yogi places his daily enema on a par with brushing his teeth. There are routines to clean the colon, stomach, and respiratory organs. As you can imagine, they are complicated and require a great deal of practice and the utmost concentration. They should never be attempted except under the supervision of an experienced instructor. I have tried some out of curiosity, but I do not practice them or advocate their practice. Not that I question their effectiveness. On the contrary, I well believe that their proper practice can assure perfect health. However, I feel that an extreme preoccupation with health, or anything else for that matter, can lead to an unhealthy fanaticism that warps the personality.

An occasional enema is beneficial and preferable to any laxative or cathartic which is harsh to the system. The only other internal cleansing technique I might recommend is to relieve a nasal cold by sniffing lukewarm water from the palm of the hand up one nostril and passing it out the other one. In general, the novice concerned with respiratory ailments will find that nasal breathing techniques, performed regularly, help clear up sinus conditions and nasal irritations, relieve headaches, and prevent colds.

I used to catch cold often, but since I have been practicing Yoga I rarely have one. My good health has helped my family stay healthier, too. You know how a cold or other contagious respiratory disorder goes from one member of a family to the next, so that someone is always sick and constantly reinfecting the others. Having even one person resistant to colds can break the cycle of contagion and help keep everyone in the family healthier.

You will discover as you progress in Yoga that you are feeling better than you have felt in years. Naturally, almost any exercise will benefit your physical condition and give you more vitality. Unlike your automobile, the human body does not wear out with use but is more likely to deteriorate from lack of use. Not only are Yoga exercises unparalleled in the thoroughness with which they condition every area of the body, but they are unique in that they exercise and condition the internal organs as well, which no other form of exercise does.

Very few people are aware of the working of their inner organs and their general anatomy. Through Yoga training you can become aware of your inner body and learn how to beneficially affect specific organs. The Yogi can feel each and every organ, gland, and muscle and keep it in excellent working condition.

Many people are never at peace with their digestive system. While not exactly ill, they are continually plagued by chronic discomforts such as constipation, flatulence, and heartburn, which they sheepishly attribute to "something I ate." They seek false relief in palliatives or symptom-masking drugs that only aggravate these disorders. Diet plays the major role, but exercise to stimulate and relax the digestive system is also necessary. Yoga exercises, especially the abdominal exercises, promote normalization and stimulate healthy functioning of the liver, spleen, kidneys, and all the organs of the digestive system without medications or laxatives. The Abdominal Lift, Cobra, Bow, and Locust work on all the organs in the viscera, stimulating the correct functioning of peristalsis. Some of these techniques don't have to be performed more than once a week for lasting benefits. I have students report to me alleviation of indigestion, constipation, heartburn, chronic gastritis, and colitis. I say that proper diet and mental relaxation through Yoga were the dominant factors in curing Herbert, one of my students who suffered from ulcers. But he swears that the abdominal exercises were solely responsible. I'll modify his claim and say they definitely helped.

Abdominal exercises can affect other areas besides the digestive system. George, who is a young seventy-five, was in perfect physical condition, thanks to Yoga, except for a prostate condition. He discovered that, after daily practice of the Abdominal Lift, the prostate gland returned to normal and a scheduled operation became unnecessary.

The inverted positions, such as the Shoulderstand and the Headstand, which are emphasized in Yoga also have multiple effects benefiting many parts of the body. With them you can help rest and strengthen your heart. The blood can flow freely into the organs and glands situated in the upper body, where the heart normally has to pump against gravity. The increased circulation to the thyroid gland stimulates its proper functioning in regulating the body's metabolism. This is an important factor in weight control and general vitality. The increased blood supply to the brain also helps dispel fatigue and promote mental alertness. Many of my senior citizen students tell me that the inverted postures of Yoga have improved their mental clarity. In the Shoulderstand, pressure is also removed from the blood vessels in the legs, minimizing the painful symptoms of varicose veins.

Many gynecologists are now coming to recognize the powers of correct exercise in improving the condition of the organs and helping to clear up gynecological disturbances. Many of the exercises these doctors recommend are identical or similar to Yoga techniques. Postpartum instructions include abdominal breathing to strengthen the abdominal muscles and inverted postures to recondition the pelvic organs after childbirth. Menstrual cramps can also be relieved with these positions. I know of one case in which practicing the Shoulderstand corrected an enlargement of the uterus and another one in which it remedied an enlarged ovary.

We teach Yoga to many women who have had radical or partial mastectomies, and to women who have suffered from degeneration of tissue in the arm. Yoga exercises have restored complete mobility and flexibility in the arm, shoulder, and surrounding areas, as well as providing a boost in morale during the difficult adjustment period.

Relaxation methods derived from Yoga are used in natural childbirth to relieve pain and help achieve an easier delivery. Yoga can also be used to help restore emotional equilibrium during the "blue days" women are prone to periodically—before a menstrual period, in postpartum depression, and during menopause. The relaxation and deep breathing can be very effectively used to alleviate the tensions accompanying menopause and menstruation, and the other exercises will help relieve the cramps and backaches many women suffer during their periods.

The Cobra, Locust, and Bow especially are known to be sexually rejuvenating for both men and women. They also affect the kidneys and the complete urinary system. One of my students suffered from chronic cystitis, a painful inflammation of the bladder which formerly could be relieved only through dilation and powerful antibiotics. She has practiced

Yoga for three years, and her condition has not flared up in two years. She attributes her improvement to all the exercises, with special emphasis on the Cobra, Locust, and Bow. I also advised her to drink fresh vegetable juices, and she considers the combination infallible.

Many who hear about my success in strengthening my back and who suffer from back conditions, arthritis, rheumatism, or other physical handicaps ask me whether they should attempt to do Yoga. I don't encourage them, because I am not medically trained. Neither do I discourage them except in cases where I know or suspect that exercise may be harmful—in extreme hypertension, certain heart conditions, or where there is the possibility of sprain, fracture, or dislocation in any part of the body.

I strongly advise them to consult a doctor before they start. Once they begin Yoga, I work with them individually as much as I can, and in the course of my teaching I have achieved some marvelous results with these kinds of problems.

Arthritis alone cripples millions of people in this country, and despite all the research being carried out, no prevention or cure has been found for it. The drugs that are offered to arthritis sufferers may partially relieve the symptoms but cannot cure the disease. In some cases these drugs produce dangerous side effects. Some doctors, especially osteopaths and chiropractors, advocate exercise. I have seen Yoga exercise help sufferers from arthritis and other rheumatoid diseases. Moreover, I am convinced that everyone has a tendency to arthritis, which can be prevented with correct exercise.

Once a person has begun to suffer the effects of arthritis, it takes a great deal of courage to exercise. Drugs are a much easier way out. However, the longer an arthritic person waits to try exercise, the more damage the disease does, until the crippling effects are so severe that it is too late for exercise to help.

The person suffering from arthritis or a similar crippling affliction should not begin any exercise program without a doctor's approval, and at the beginning he must be extremely careful. There is no better exercise than Yoga for these cases, because it is so gentle and gradual.

Rita was one of my students determined to help herself with exercise. She was in great pain because of arthritis, in spite of cortisone injections, but wanted to try Yoga—she had tried everything else. In the beginning, it was painful to sense her pain as she attempted even the simplest movement. But as time went on, it became enormously gratifying to watch her improvement from week to week. Slowly but obviously, the joints relaxed as the blood was allowed to flow naturally through the body. Today she can perform all basic Yoga positions without pain and has regained complete flexibility. Rose, another arthritis sufferer, who won't reveal her age but is probably around sixty-five, started Yoga a few months ago and already is experiencing a new lease on life because of the improvement in her condition.

Then there is Arlene, who had had polio at thirteen. She had conquered the crippling effects, but was left with complete rigidity of all muscles and joints, especially in the back area. She also happens to be a professional singer. She has so benefited from Yoga that recently when she auditioned for a singing role that also required her to dance, she was chosen for the part.

The way those people feel was summed up by one of my students whose bursitis disappeared after three months of Yoga. "It's a miracle!" she said. "No," I told her. "It was no miracle. You did it yourself with hard work."

One ailment that the American public is becoming increasingly concerned about is heart disease. Justifiably so, for heart and vascular ailments claim more than a million victims a year. Physicians are prescribing exercise as the best way to prevent heart attacks and even advising some of those with existing heart conditions to exercise. The trend is toward vigorous exercise, particularly jogging. Jogging, however, is not good for everyone. I think it is excellent to begin if you are young or in first-class physical condition. But certainly no one past thirty-five or forty should start out on such a strenuous activity without a medical okay. A California survey a few years ago reported that there have been a number of deaths resulting from jogging. Presumably these people had had no preliminary medical examination or professional supervision of their jogging programs.

In our sedentary society, where the automobile is used even for an errand to the nearest corner, it would seem more logical to make people walk, at a vigorous pace, that is, before turning them loose to jog. Next to Yoga and swimming, the finest exercise is walking. It conditions the entire body without undue strain. But walking is becoming obsolete. My husband and I live in a quiet suburban neighborhood, ideal for walking, yet we are the only people who ever take walks in the area. I'm sure the neighbors regard us as eccentrics because of our strange habit of walking.

Any exercise started at an early age can be pursued throughout a lifetime without extra strain on the body. Anyone at age eighty who has played tennis, bicycled, or ice skated all his life can maintain his health and energy by continuing these activities. But it is only common sense that someone without previous training, unaccustomed to exercise, who suddenly begins tennis, handball, basketball, vigorous calisthenics, or running becomes an excellent candidate for an early heart attack.

Yoga can be started at any age without strain. The slow, gradual movements build up energy without depleting the existing supply of it. Never forcing, never straining the body builds its endurance by stretching to its capacity, holding the stretch, and progressing to increased capacity. The breathing exercises, performed by themselves and in conjunction with the positions, increase the supply of oxygen to the blood, naturally stimulating the heart. Doctors have recommended Yoga to combat the tension and stress which lie at the root of so many heart disorders. The part that Yoga plays in controlling weight and discouraging smoking and the consumption of alcohol adds to its benefits in keeping your heart healthy.

Yoga knows no age limit. I have students in my classes in their sixties and seventies who, because of Yoga, have more physical vigor than people half their age. As a group they suffer less from the ailments that are so common among old people, discomforts like constipation, muscular stiffness, and low resistance to respiratory infections. Yoga also helps prevent arteriosclerosis, or hardening of the arteries, often suffered by the aged. It is, of course, much better to begin maintaining a healthy body with exercise in youth rather than trying to regain health in old age. But it is never too late to start Yoga. Because Yoga exercises are non-strenuous, older people can find a plan of exercise which is feasible to carry out without undue fatigue. When it comes to the aging process, Yoga cannot stop the clock, but it can slow it down. The Yogis have shown that old age does not have to be a time of feebleness, sickness, and depression, as it usually is with elderly people. Inactivity and the discouraged attitude that accompanies it accelerate the aging process. Yoga exercises decelerate and, in some cases, even reverse the process by increasing vitality, restoring flexibility, promoting the healthy functioning of organs and glands, improving blood circulation, controlling weight, and firming muscles. In addition, they help relieve the nervous tension suffered by the elderly.

The people who receive the greatest Yoga benefits unconsciously are the hypochondriacs, with whom I sympathize, because at one time I was one of them. They are the ones who start the course with a long list of aches and pains. Every week they tell me of another ill effect from the previous lesson. Then their bodies start to respond to Yoga with a wonderful feeling of well-being, and the day comes when all of a sudden nothing whatever hurts them. If I confront them with this change, they look at me blankly and say that naturally they feel fine and have always felt fine.

The best cure for any sickness is prevention, and the best insurance for good health in middle and old age is learning how to care for the body in youth. Flexibility is no problem with little children, but it is surprising how much of that natural resiliency has already been lost by the time they become teen-agers. Nevertheless, their bodies are generally still pliable enough to get very fast results with Yoga, an advantage that makes it attractive to the impatient nature of the adolescent. Yoga is ideal for the teen-ager in many other respects. It attacks the problems that beset most teen-agers—overweight, poor complexion, and gawkiness—by helping to control weight, stimulating proper circulation, and improving coordination and poise. In addition, the relaxation and breathing techniques help the adolescent better handle his emotions. They also improve his powers of concentration.

Physical fitness is stressed in schools today more than previously; however, the curriculum of many elementary schools still does not include a physical education program but features only lukewarm exercises chosen by the classroom teacher. I have quite a few teachers in my classes who recognize the need for a physical program that teaches the children overall exercises that condition every part of the body. Some of these teachers have undertaken to teach Yoga exercises to their grade-school charges, and they report an enthusiastic response from the children. One of them plans to teach Yoga in summer camp this year. Another of my very dedicated teacher-students wants to try teaching it to brain-damaged children, and I am helping her plan a program.

Physical educators, especially in Europe, advocate that an exercise program begin at kindergarten age in order to lay the foundation for good health in adulthood, for what is instilled in the young child will be followed in later life. Physical education programs in our schools emphasize games and sports that most people cannot or do not care to continue as adults. It's a rare housewife who pursues volleyball to keep in shape.

If you ever practice when your children are around, you'll see how eager they'll be to try the exercises, too. Because they're so flexible, they'll be able to do them quite easily. If you're going to become demoralized watching your daughter assume the Lotus posture at first try, while you're still trying to get your own knee to touch the floor, don't let her see you practice your Yoga until you've mastered a few of the positions. Teaching Yoga to children as part of their physical education will provide them with a practical method to maintain flexibility and good health all their lives.

9

YOGA
AND
SEX

To IMMEDIATELY SQUELCH the rumors about sex and Yoga, let me assure you that you don't have to give up the first when you take up the second. One common misconception is that chastity is essential to the successful practice of Yoga. Some Indian Yogis, Swamis, and Gurus do maintain that only the celibate can wholeheartedly devote himself to the study of the more advanced positions, breathing exercises, and meditation. They believe that true spirituality can be achieved only by those freed from sexual drives. There is no denying that sex and marriage certainly do take up one's energy and time. Without the responsibilities of family life, you could become more proficient in Yoga by being able to practice whenever you wanted to without outside distractions. As far as I know,

none of the religious saints were ever married. Understandably so, for it would be a difficult task to become a saint when
one had to earn a living for a family and contend with a
demanding spouse and noisy children. But leaving the wife
and kids doesn't make one a saint, nor does abstinence from
sexual intercourse make one spiritual. As a rule, the person
who equates sexual intercourse with spiritual defilement is
hiding his own psychological problems behind a shield of
distorted virtue.

The association of sexual abstinence with Yoga is fostered
by the fanatic Hindu followers of Yoga. The sexual life of the
Hindu is a continual struggle against contradictions. His own
sexual drives, constantly stimulated, are in direct conflict
with his society's view that the ideal Hindu is chaste. His
family life is by turn indulgent, severe, and restrictive, with
the woman occupying a degraded position in it. The role of
the Hindu woman represents failure from the day she is
born, because she should have been a son. Married off by her
parents at an early age, as a wife she continues in her inferior
role, even among the upper classes, becoming a servant to her
husband, trotting humbly behind him, eating only after he
has finished, and generally being banned from male society.
The primitive idea still prevails that a woman is unclean
during menstruation and for a time after childbirth.

Regarded as a passive, servile cow, her one purpose is to
bear sons. It is only with the birth of a son that the Hindu
woman is raised from her lowly position. This is her season of
exaltation, for since the father does not want to be bothered
with the messy aspects of raising children during their early
years, the mother is completely in charge. As a baby and
young child, the Indian son is pampered, coddled, and
smothered in mother love. He is nursed to a standing-up age
and often sleeps with his mother until the age of ten or twelve.
This type of mother-son relationship in Western society has

been proven to be harmful to the child, conducive to homosexuality, and at the very least a hindrance to his chances for a healthy sexual relationship when he is an adult.

When the son is about ten or twelve the father steps in, wielding his authority with an iron hand, and rules the lives of his children until the day he dies. Even after the son marries, he is still treated as a child, expected to defer to his father's wishes.

In his autobiography Gandhi writes that he was expected not even to converse with his bride in his father's presence, as if by ignoring her, the girl and his own sexual role as her husband could be willed out of existence.

Another important factor shaping the Hindu's sexual attitude is the belief that man's vital energy is concentrated in his seminal fluid, stored in a cavity in his skull. Every orgasm depletes him of his physical and spiritual powers. This belief often leads to an obsessive preoccupation with preserving the semen, preferably by preventing discharge through total abstinence from masturbation and sexual intercourse. Some who succumb to the temptations of the flesh go through involved maneuvers to prevent ejaculation during intercourse or to bring the discharged semen back into their bodies. Obviously, this practice is not widespread and is too difficult for general birth control.

Tantric Yoga is deemed to be the highest Yoga, said to supersede Jnana Yoga of the intellect. Much has been written about it, but it is practiced only by a very few, because it is the most difficult of all Yogas to achieve. It is the sexual act of lovemaking without culmination or orgasm. It involves the holding back of orgasm in order to recycle energy instead of releasing it and in order to rise from the physical act to spiritual levels. The advocates of Tantric Yoga claim that it is the expression of pure love and true relaxation in the sex act, and that the relaxation instead of the ejaculation becomes the total fulfillment. There is only love play without time limitations, and all its sensations can be truly savored. It means truly relating to another person and his or her needs and pleasures, leading to higher meditation and possibly Samadhi.

It sounds very beautiful, but it has many drawbacks. First you must find a willing partner, and you both must have unlimited time to practice, which means you must for that time actually forego all other activities. It seems very confusing that Tantric Yoga is supposedly life-giving and life-restoring, yet completely ignores procreation. On the surface it appears to be very much oriented to the woman. The female partner can indulge in limitless foreplay; she takes the top position in the sex act and directs the action, and she may have all the orgasms she wants without the fear of pregnancy. What Tantric Yoga really comes down to, when you wade through all the flowery language, is the prolongation of the male's lifespan through preservation of sperm.

I personally believe that Tantric Yoga is pure male chauvinism and that it originated from the concept that the sex act is physically and spiritually degrading to the man, that the woman is the temptress and the aggressor, for in all the Tantric erotic pictures and sculptures, the man's expression can lead one to believe that he is merely an innocent bystander in the depicted sexual goings-on.

Ironically, the Indians' way of life is geared to incite sexual stimulation. In most aspects they are prudish and mid-Victorian in their sexual attitudes. Yet it is a land abounding in phallic-symbol cults, sex-charged mythology, temples with sculptures and paintings which graphically display unbelievably intricate variations of the sex act, and merchants doing an unrivalled trade in aphrodisiacs. Also, the spicy food the Indian favors, his everyday consumption of hot peppers and strong curries, increases his sexual appetite. All in all, his environment intensifies his sexual dilemma.

To the Indian, simultaneously stimulated and repressed,

the ideal and envied man is the Yogi, who experiences no loss of his precious seminal fluids, who can abjure sex altogether, and is, therefore, rewarded with magical powers, such as the ability to become invisible or to levitate himself. This last, of course, is fiction, but it is true that the Yogi can control his sex urges and desires. Through constant practice of external and internal Yoga exercises, he can regulate the function of every part of his body, every muscle, gland, and inner organ. He can direct the action of the thyroid and pituitary glands, the muscle in his penis, and control his erection. Meditation and the ability to regulate his breathing enable him to master his emotions as well. And his great emotional control in turn further restrains his physical urges. The Yogi's diet also contributes to his sexual self-control, for he foregoes rich, overly seasoned, spicy foods in favor of bland, non-stimulating foods.

But although the Yogi is in charge of his sexual impulses, he neither suppresses them nor denies their existence. Yoga does not impose chastity, celibacy, or continence, because that would be in opposition to the laws of nature. To go against nature is wrong. On the other hand, regarding sex as a natural function is not equivalent to license. Copulation is not like taking a drink of water when you're thirsty, for man is on a higher level than animals, and so necessarily should be his mating habits. Yoga advocates the exercise of discrimination and control in sexual activities, as in other activities, to achieve self-realization. In sexual intercourse with someone he loves, man can use his body to attain spiritual and physical bliss.

Sex is very much a part of Yoga symbolism, a most obvious example being the legend of Kundalini already mentioned. The serpent is used as a sexual symbol in the early folklore of all peoples, as for instance in the story of Adam and Eve in the Garden of Eden, where the snake's introduction of carnal knowledge led to their expulsion from Paradise. By contrast, in the Yoga Kundalini legend the height of self-realization is reached with the union of male and female. Here is the difference between the Western and Yoga attitudes toward sex. Western teachings say sex is bad, a weakness of the flesh which is to be denied. Yoga recognizes the tremendous force of sexual energy as part of man's total energy to be utilized in his quest for self-realization.

Yoga does not try to repress man's sexual drive, because it realizes how damaging sexual repression is. Everywhere in the world, except maybe among remote aboriginal tribes, sex has evolved from a natural and pleasurable function into an intense moral and psychological problem. After more than a hundred years of Victorian repression, the United States is being rocked with a sexual explosion. We are bombarded with sex in advertising, books, movies, and plays. The fear of pregnancy, the club once used to keep "nice" girls from indulging in sex, has been eliminated with the Pill. Suddenly our society has awakened to SEX and doesn't seem to know how to cope with it.

Much could be learned from Yoga, which channels sexual energy and directs it into other creative areas. The Yogi sublimates his sexual drives into other outlets for his own benefit and often for the benefit of society. Freud made it clear how the individual turned his sexual drives into other areas of activity. Thus, the spinster, with no children of her own, could find an outlet for her emotions as a teacher or nurse. The Yogi who has retreated to the monastic life is celibate without effort or denial, for all his energies are devoted to the rigors of advanced Yoga. But there are also those Yogis who are householders, fulfilling their role as husbands and using their knowledge of Yoga to enhance their sexual life.

Basic Yoga teachings are concerned with the establishment of a satisfactory sex life for physical and mental health. Yoga can increase sexual pleasure in many ways. It can be instrumental in changing an inhibiting attitude, for Yoga contains none of the prudishness toward the body and its natural functions that has been an integral part of Western culture for so long. The way one feels about sex plays a subtle but real part in the ability to enjoy its pleasures. Sampling the current best sellers and movies should convince anyone that society is certainly becoming more open about sex and nudity, but the very manner in which four-letter words and bare bosoms are flaunted indicates that an intelligent, mature attitude has not yet been attained. Even the generation of people now in their twenties and early thirties, with all their emphasis on sexual freedom, still react to the ideas they were taught as children, that there is something dirty about sex. In my opinion it will take at least two more generations to outgrow these notions. The sex education now being introduced into the curriculum of many school systems, if it is presented intelligently, can help society arrive at a healthy sexual attitude.

In any successful personal relationship there must be a balance of give and take. If one person is selfish and inconsiderate, the other person becomes resentful and hurt, and the relationship suffers. Nowhere is this situation more intense than in the marriage bed. A husband intent only on his own gratification often leaves his wife unsatisfied. In time she may become cool to his demands; he may then regard her as unresponsive, aggravating the problems in their relationship even more, and this situation very often leads to divorce. As I have said before, the practice of Yoga exerts a subtle change on the personality. As you continue, you will become more patient and understanding toward other people. These qualities will carry over into your sexual life, and as you become more concerned for your partner's gratification, you will evoke a responsiveness that will add to your mutual pleasures.

However, not all sexual problems are based on psychological causes, as used to be generally assumed. More and more, current scientific investigations are attributing sexual inadequacies to physical causes. With some sexually indifferent or incompetent people the problem may be glandular. These people often find that Yoga exercises reawaken their sexual desire and improve their ability to perform the sex act. Many Yoga postures were deliberately designed to stimulate the sexual appetite and correct sluggishly functioning endocrine glands, which include parts of the gonads or sex glands. The Plough and the Locust are two of the best exercises for stimulating the gonads. The inverted postures such as the Headstand, Shoulderstand, and Camel improve the functioning of the pituitary gland, the master gland influencing most basic physical functions. Glandular problems affecting sexual performance can be corrected in a short time by practicing Yoga holds and positions.

Yoga also acts as an equalizer, for while it stimulates the sexual appetite and awakens dormant desires, at the same time it teaches control of sexual urges.

As a rule, my male students don't discuss their sexual problems or relate their improvements to me or to the class, but they can't help dropping veiled remarks or disguise their joy in their achievements. Yoga practice can stabilize man's control of his erection and correct premature ejaculation, a common source of unhappiness in marriage. The increased ability to restrain ejaculation, which can be gained through Yoga, leads to the adjustments necessary to conform to the woman's slower achievement of her climax.

A woman who couldn't experience an orgasm was once usually directed to psychotherapy, where she'd try to work through her problem or learn to adjust to it. However, now doctors know that the cause of frigidity is very often muscular. Improving the vaginal-urinary muscle tone by contracting these muscles can help increase a woman's pleasure during sexual intercourse.

Although many of the Yoga exercises benefit the gonads, remember the sex glands do not lead a separate existence. They are part of your body and are affected by the general condition of your body just as the digestive system is. A person who keeps his body in peak condition through Yoga will lead a healthy, vital life and as a result can also enjoy an active, satisfying sex life for many years. Masters and Johnson have stressed the importance of good health for effective sexual functioning. They have also cited fatigue and tension among the most common causes of sexual failure. With the Yoga exercises and breathing you can effectively combat these two deterrents to successful sexual activity.

No list of the ways Yoga helps to achieve a happy sexual life would be complete without reminding you that Yoga exercises can give you a more desirable body. And after all, being attractive to a partner is the first step on the road to sexual happiness. Confidence in your own body also helps get rid of inhibitions.

There are Yoga teachers who work with specific sex problems, but I personally teach Yoga for the overall benefit rather than stressing solutions to particular problems. Therefore most of my students start Yoga completely unaware of these particular benefits, yet many of them report the favorable ways that Yoga has affected their sexual experiences. One of my students, whom I will call Betty, told me that her inability to experience an orgasm had cost her many hours in analysis discussing her problem and many more hours worrying about it with her husband. After three months of Yoga practice, she reached her first orgasm. From then on she and her husband began experiencing a mutually gratifying sex life. Another student, who after the birth of her fourth child developed an aversion to sex—one of the Pill's occasional side effects—in spite of the "insurance" against pregnancy, found that her former healthy enjoyment of sexual intercourse returned with intensive Yoga practice. The wife of a man who had become seriously interested in Yoga told me that when he was fifty his sex urges had dwindled to zero, but at fifty-five he had become a new man, full of vigor in the marital bed. Many men who think they've reached the age of impotency find that Yoga can rejuvenate them.

One of my young married students shared this experience with me. Her husband, who had not expressed any interest in learning Hatha Yoga, but who is very limber and agile, wandered into the bedroom as she was practicing her exercises along with my tape recording. He joined her in the hour of practice and in the ensuing relaxation, and they began their lovemaking in a truly relaxed state of mind and body. She relates that each had total awareness of the other and of their bodies, a deep rather than a fierce passion. The time factor was forgotten and orgasm for both of them was almost like a religious experience.

If two partners can learn to practice the Yoga positions and the breathing techniques together and can help and direct each other with them, it can help their sex life become truly beautiful and meaningful.

In contrast to Tantric Yoga, which urges total repression of the orgasm, Hatha Yoga can lead to orgasms that are totally fulfilling for both partners, not limited to the genital area, but rather encompassing the entire body and psyche. Orgasm in our present day has become such a social and mental hang-up that all the preoccupation with it must surely be taking some of the pleasure out of sex. Is she getting enough? Am I getting enough? Is it adequate, rich enough, well-timed? Instead of a natural event, for many sex has turned into a competitive battle and cause for divorce.

When two people are in contact and harmony, they can approach the sex act physically and mentally relaxed. There is excitement, yes, and pleasure—but no compulsion, no frenzy, no force. The mind is centered not on climax, but on total enjoyment with each other in each other, and when the orgasm comes about, it provides a total release of tensions instead of having only a temporary effect.

Grim determination to enjoy sex is self-defeating. Learn to relax, with Yoga. As tension subsides, the benefits manifest themselves. Sexual stimulation, sexual control, and the ingredients for a happy and harmonious sex life can evolve naturally through Yoga.

10

YOGA
AND
SMOKING

To the compulsive smoker Yoga offers a way to stop. I will tell you how. I don't have to tell you why. Ever since 1964, when the Surgeon General's Report on Smoking and Health warned that cigarette smoking was a health hazard, statistics have been piling up linking cigarettes with not only cancer and heart disease but a whole list of other disorders, including emphysema, sinus trouble, bronchitis, ulcers, arthritis, and migraine. However, in spite of the mounting evidence that smoking will shorten your life, millions continue to smoke. It seems that the older generation has stopped smoking to a degree, but this decrease is balanced off by young people, who now smoke more than ever. At various times, anti-smoking laws are enforced in public buildings, institutions, and schools, but generally they do not seem to have had a great effect. In spite of the increasingly high cost of tobacco and the warning on the cigarette packs: "The Surgeon General Has Determined That Cigarette Smoking Is Dangerous to Your Health," the cigarette industry is not suffering any fall in revenues at all.

In the past the smoker confronted with the question, "Why do you smoke?" could glibly answer, "Because I enjoy it." But in view of the fact that the smoker is shortening his own life, that kind of rationalization just doesn't stand up. Why, then, does he smoke? Because he can't stop.

I am aware that there were lots of smokers who read the articles on the dangers of smoking and said, "That's it. I'm kicking the habit, starting now." And they were successful. Because for some smokers smoking constitutes just that—a habit that can be licked with a modicum of effort. But for others, I contend that smoking is an addiction, as surely as the compulsive use of alcohol and drugs is an addiction. Like any addiction, it is a psychological and physiological sickness that puts the afflicted at the mercy of his compulsion, sometimes forcing him to sacrifice even his dignity and self-respect.

This was illustrated very vividly for me in Germany after World War II, when GI cigarettes became currency. A carton of cigarettes, purchased at the PX for $1.50, could be sold for as much as $100 on the black market. Jewels, heirlooms—and hard to believe, but true—mothers, sisters, and daughters were sold for cigarettes. Any GI smoking in the street would attract a following of Germans who would fight like vultures over his discarded stub.

And what else but an addiction could compel intelligent people to continue after their doctors have specifically warned them they are courting death by smoking? Even an intellectual giant like Sigmund Freud suffered and died from cancer of the mouth and throat caused by excessive cigar smoking.

Another characteristic that marks smoking as an addiction is the painful withdrawal symptoms the chain smoker experiences when his system is deprived of nicotine: dizziness, nausea, headaches, vomiting, tremors, mental depression, and anxiety.

I am very much aware of what it means to be a cigarette addict because I used to be one. I started smoking at seventeen, when I was living with relatives. They gave me strict instructions never to smoke. Resenting them, I began smoking as a means of getting back at them. To a youngster a cigarette can be a psychological symbol of all his desires and frustrations, his rebellion, his yearnings for social status, acceptance, and maturity.

During the many years I smoked, sometimes as many as sixty cigarettes a day, I felt guilty and desperately wanted to stop. I only remember two days during that time when I did not smoke. One was when I had my tonsils removed (I smoked the next day), and the other was the day of the accident, when I was semi-conscious and couldn't move. I smoked up to my last labor pain, and when I opened my eyes, I reached for a cigarette before asking about the baby. How well I remember the panic-stricken hunts through all purses and pockets in the house for a cigarette and the 2:00 A.M. drives to find an open drugstore when I had run out. There was nothing I could do without being fortified by a cigarette from the time I awoke, sleepily groping for a pack, until I went to sleep. I was an addict; I learned to live with the fact that, like the alcoholic, if I ever took "just one more," I'd be hooked again.

Yoga enabled me to stop smoking, because it operates on the addiction on many levels. You don't *have* to be an addict to stop smoking with Yoga. Yoga will make it easier for any kind of smoker to kick his habit, but to the addict it will be a life saver.

It may sound as if I'm contradicting myself when I tell you not to go into Yoga to stop smoking. You can't grit your teeth and jump into Yoga as you would into a cold bath. The idea that This Is Going To Be Good For Me If It Kills Me just won't work with Yoga—not even to accomplish a goal as beneficial as giving up smoking. There is no pressure in Yoga to accomplish a goal. If you bring that kind of tension to Yoga, you nullify its results. Nothing can be forced in Yoga. Begin Yoga because you will enjoy it. All the benefits come naturally, including the desire and steadfastness to give up smoking. Yoga can succeed where other methods have failed, because it is an effective substitute for smoking.

Several times in my smoking years, I went through all sorts of antics to give up cigarettes. The first time I tried to quit I formed a no-smoking partnership with my sister-in-law. How proud we were when we announced to the world that we had smoked our last cigarette. We spent hours on the phone comparing symptoms and encouraging each other. And we ate and ate and ate. My freedom from nicotine lasted four months—until the day we went shopping for dresses, because neither of us could fit into any of our clothes. We both discovered we had increased our girth by two dress sizes. We tried to laugh at ourselves in our outsize dresses, but the laughter wasn't very sincere. I went back to cigarettes. (My sister-in-law stuck it out, gained up to fifty pounds during the next two years, and only began to take off the weight when I introduced her to Yoga.)

After I had had my brief taste of a cigarette-free life, the thought of stopping never left me. I knew I needed a substitute, and I next turned to chewing gum. Every time I had the urge for a cigarette, I would pop a piece of gum into my mouth, turning from a chain smoker into a chain chewer. When I next visited my dentist, the condition of my teeth and gums was so bad he warned me that if I continued chewing gum I wouldn't have any teeth left. As a sacrifice to dental health, I lit up again. There were other attempts to quit with other substitutes like tranquilizers and commercial medicines—all just as harmful and inadequate.

Sound familiar? Of course, because many people go through much the same motions to stop smoking. And they fail, as I did, because in most cases they want to fail. They want to prove it can't be done. They would *like* to stop smoking, but they don't really *want* to give it up, because they cannot face a permanently smokeless existence.

They would never stop feeling sorry for themselves for being deprived of their need. Giving up smoking permanently can only work when the person is ready to accept the new freedom from nicotine joyfully instead of dejectedly. That is why the substitute for smoking must prove satisfying and represent purpose. Yoga is that kind of substitute.

Yoga will train your body and mind to want to stop smoking. When you begin the Yoga breathing exercises, you will be bringing more air into your lungs than they have known for years. As you continue and begin to master the breathing exercises, you will feel your lungs clearing up, nasal congestion relieved, and your throat no longer feeling like the proverbial inside of a motorman's glove. You won't be so anxious to light up and lose that country fresh-air feeling—the real thing, not the mentholated taste advertised in certain brands of cigarettes. With the increased supply of oxygen in the system, the desire to smoke is killed.

The other exercises, too, will begin to have their effect on your body, providing you with a new sense of physical well-being that you won't want to lose by smoking. Gradually your body will begin to reject cigarettes. The more engrossed in

Yoga you become, the stronger will be your desire to stop. As you gain proficiency in the various positions, you will be spurred on to work toward the more complex holds. You'll discover the effects of smoking are actually an obstacle to your performance. Pride in your achievements will begin tipping the scales against smoking. You will realize that Yoga and smoking are physically incompatible. From then, it is merely a matter of time until you decide to do without cigarettes.

Yoga also works on the tension that many people claim is their reason for smoking. Actually, it is mostly the smoking that causes the tension that cigarettes are supposedly being used to relieve. Yoga helps eliminate the tension, no matter how it is caused. Because the exercises act as a relaxant, you can begin to lose tension before you stop smoking. With less tension in your system, you feel less need to smoke. As you smoke less, you will find you are experiencing even less tension and therefore are not so likely to use a cigarette as a tranquilizer. As with so many other effects of Yoga, the process is a circular one, with your body and Yoga working together for your benefit.

When you first quit smoking, you will experience that old familiar yen for a cigarette. The commonest ploy for coping with that reaction is to put something else in the mouth—usually something loaded with calories. When the desire for a cigarette inevitably returns, in goes another hard candy, candy bar, martini, bag of potato chips, and so on up to twenty pounds. I think the most frequent excuse for not giving up smoking might be the three little words, "I'll get fat." Well, oxygen doesn't contain a single calorie, and that's what Yoga teaches you to use with great effectiveness in annihilating that recurrent yen for a cigarette. You're able to give up smoking without the aid of gum, candy, liquor, or other fattening "foods."

When you get the urge to smoke, practice the breathing exercises. You can do the Complete Breath without raising your shoulders and the Abdominal Breath anywhere—at the office, the PTA meeting, the check-out line at the supermarket—without anyone noticing. The rhythmic breathing will suppress the desire for a cigarette. The forceful breathing of the Bellows Breath, which you will probably prefer to do in private, will get rid of the poisonous tobacco pollution that has settled on the walls of your lungs. As time goes on, the urge to smoke will disturb you less and less frequently. Gradually, the effects of the exercises and breathing practiced in your regular exercise period will be carried over during the day.

Once you've joined the ranks of nonsmokers, you'll be able to stay there. The mind and body will once more become used to their natural condition of doing without cigarettes. Other pleasures will begin to compensate for not smoking: better health, more pep, a sharper sense of taste and smell, and an improvement in your looks. Let me warn you, though, the desire to smoke may still creep up on you, even long after you've given it up. But your firmness of purpose will enable you to control that desire. If it persists, a few Yoga breaths will banish it. Because of Yoga you will be stronger than the desire to smoke.

I have a gentlemen's agreement with the smokers in my class: they don't admit it, and I don't question them. I can detect it, of course, at their first deep inhalation. Many of them started the course because they suffered from shortness of breath, wheezing, sinus conditions, or perpetual colds. Even they begin to breathe better in spite of their smoking. Harry was one of the confirmed chain smokers who had started Yoga for the fun of it. But, to his great surprise, he took to it as a duck to water. He was about thirty-five years old with a good, but stiff, body. As his back became more flexible, he was able to try and master the most intricate Yoga exercises. Once he discovered that smoking interfered with the hold of the positions he tapered off (he was one of the few who could) and eventually quit. He admitted to me that he had always wanted to stop smoking, but had never known how to go about it.

For many, Yoga has been the way to go about it. Yoga can provide you with the incentive, means, and firmness of purpose to stop smoking forever.

11

YOGA
AND
INTELLIGENT
NUTRITION

GOOD NUTRITION is the foundation on which all good health is built. The guiding principles of the Yogi tell him to eat what can benefit him and not to eat what can harm him. Anyone can use these same principles of Yoga for good nutrition once he has learned what these beneficial and harmful foods are. Most people, if they give any thought at all to the nutritional value of their diet, are misled by the fallacy that they can indulge themselves in anything edible so long as they eat some of the good stuff, too. But eating the right food cannot prevent the harm done to the body by eating the wrong food. In nutrition, as in medicine, that ounce of prevention is worth a pound of cure.

Malnutrition in America is an unfortunate fact of life. It is indeed shameful that in the United States distressed areas exist where people suffer from malnutrition because of poverty. But national surveys have also revealed that malnutrition is not exclusively a problem of the poor. Those who involuntarily suffer from inadequate diets are a relative handful compared to the millions who create their own nutritional deficiencies in the midst of plenty. Although it seems ludicrous that the citizens of a nation with our abundant resources should suffer from malnutrition, there is no doubt that we do so *because* of that very affluence. Not only do we stuff ourselves with too much food, but no other nation consumes as much devitalized, denatured, overprocessed, synthetic food as we do. Money alone does not alleviate malnutrition; it does, in fact, aggravate it.

Generally speaking, we eat advertising copy instead of food. We allow ourselves to be mesmerized by the commercial hucksters who lull us into false security about the nutritional values of packaged, frozen and canned foods which we have the money to buy. We are the prey of the powerful food industries, which hire the advertisers and continue to manufacture unhealthful, unnutritional, poisonous and expensive foodstuffs. We are told of the dangers of consuming health-hazardous foods, yet we find every possible excuse— "Our government really wouldn't allow us to be poisoned"; "It can't be bad if it's advertised"; "Everyone else is eating it"; "You've got to eat something."

In my opinion, it is imperative that public education be instituted, starting in the grade schools, to educate people to choose proper foods and to reject improper foods. Our hospitals are filled with victims of faulty nutrition, who suffer from chronic and degenerative diseases such as diabetes, arthritis, heart conditions, ulcers, and cancer, all caused or aggravated by eating too much of the wrong foods. Ironically, people are put on proper diets when these conditions have become acute—when it is often too late.

Many times digestive problems are danger signals that something is wrong with the organism as a whole, but too often these symptoms are camouflaged with antacids and alkalizers instead of being investigated and remedied by sensible diet. Certainly the stress they place on wholesome food is a major reason for the unusually fine health enjoyed by Yogis and dedicated students of Yoga. Americans could find no better guide to the choosing of proper food than the nutritional principles of Yoga.

The prevailing public misconception is that if one is a Yogi or serious Yoga student one's diet consists solely of sunflower seeds, tiger's milk, soy-bean products, kelp, and similar foodstuffs, and one patronizes the health-food stores for all subsistence. This is not so. Yoga teachings are primarily concerned with the freshness and cleanliness of food. With a few exceptions, most foods which meet Yoga standards can be bought in any good food store.

Misinformed Yoga fans and health-food faddists also proclaim that good health can be achieved only with organically grown food. They point out that we are being poisoned *en masse* by the chemical fertilizers and insecticides used on commercially grown food. Because of this problem, it seems that anything sells if it is labeled organic, be it food, vitamins or soap. I have my own personal doubts about some of the products claiming to be organic. The only way to be absolutely positive that you are getting real organically grown food is by growing it in your own backyard.

I don't deny that our food is subjected to chemical poisons, nor do I dispute the fact that we are victims of pollution. However, people obsessed with eating *only* organically grown products are to me in the same category as those who build their own atom-bomb shelters—they may be the only survivors when everyone else is wiped out, but they will be terribly lonely. If you can buy organically grown foods without too much trouble or expense, by all means do so, because

it is much healthier. Also, organically grown fruit and vegetables and organically fed chickens and the eggs they lay are
more flavorful.

But while the danger of pollution through our food is a real
one, the fact is that the few particles of poisons we swallow
involuntarily will not affect us extensively in this generation,
unless our bodies are run down by disease and malnutrition,
just as a cold will more easily take hold on a run-down body.
That is why Yoga is a most effective weapon with which to
fight the menaces to health. The harmful effects of toxins and
irritants can be guarded against by keeping the body, especially the organs of elimination and detoxication, in excellent
condition. The way to achieve this is by practicing the exercises and breathing techniques, avoiding harmful stimulants,
and eating nutritional foods. There are also certain commonsense precautions we can take that make it very difficult for
harmful chemicals to affect us, such as thoroughly washing
fruits and vegetables with a brush and peeling them when we
know the skin has been heavily sprayed, as in the case of
cucumbers, for instance.

Since the present influence of the Orient has been making
its impact on Western culture, Oriental diets have also become fashionable. The most prominent of these is the Zen
macrobiotic diet, or Japanese brown-rice diet, as it is better
known. Many people ask me whether I am macrobiotic, for
they associate and confuse Yoga with Zen Buddhism. Although similarities exist, and Zen allegedly developed as a
branch of Yoga, they are not the same, and the macrobiotic
diet is far removed from the Yogic way of eating. Macrobiotic
does not refer only to eating, it is a way of thinking and a way
of living. Supposedly, it can prevent and cure any disease,
which may very well be true. It prohibits eating many foods
we are accustomed to, with emphasis on eggplant, tomatoes,
and potatoes, which are strictly taboo. Since I adore those
three foods, I personally have little interest in macrobiotic

teachings. It is, of course, a matter of more than doing without eggplant. To study and comprehend the intricacies of this science is a lifelong undertaking for the Oriental. For the Westerner, true adherence is extremely complicated, not only because of the philosophy, but because some of the required foods are almost impossible to obtain anywhere but in the East. Many food fanatics follow the diet haphazardly, sometimes with tragic results, as in the case of one woman whose death was attributed to eating brown rice exclusively.

That is why many ignorant people have labeled this diet dangerous. On the same kind of distorted evidence, people who don't understand Yoga accuse it of being dangerous. I was confronted with this charge by a physician, who told me about two young girls he had treated. They had taken up Yoga and become dangerously ill, he said. As he elaborated on his accusation, it turned out that it was not Yoga but the ignorance of the girls that was to blame. These girls believed that when you take up Yoga, you must become a vegetarian. They further interpreted "vegetarian" to mean eating vegetables to the exclusion of everything else, which they did for a long time. Naturally they developed sicknesses caused by vitamin deficiency.

Although Yoga is slowly coming into its own as a modern down-to-earth way to good health, there is still much mysticism surrounding it, supported mostly by those young people who are searching for "meaning outside this hemisphere." They somehow link weird diets with Yoga.

As for vegetarianism: the concept that vegetarianism is a fundamental precept of Yoga is erroneous. Yogic writings, as such, contain no dogma either anti-carnivorous or pro-vegetarian. Vegetarianism is associated with Yoga because of its Hindu practitioners, for most sects of Hinduism forbid the slaughtering of animals. Surprisingly, many Hindu practitioners of Yoga, while they would be offended by so much as the mention of the word "meat," have no apparent objection to the ingestion of all kinds of junk foods. Others, not Hindus, believe in vegetarianism as a purely personal credo distinct from any religious affiliation. These people, who consider it morally wrong to kill an animal for food or clothing, will not eat any form of animal flesh or wear a fur coat. There are some who will eat eggs, some only eggs that have not been fertilized, and some no eggs whatsoever. There are also some vegetarians who won't eat or drink dairy products.

The true Yogi does not consider vegetarianism in itself essential to a spiritual life; nor does he consider eating meat *per se* unholy. The Yogi does, however, classify foods as either *sattvic* or *rajasic*. Sattvic is interpreted as clean, light food that is easily digestible, agreeable to the eye and palate, and soothing to the stomach. In contrast, rajasic foods are heavy, difficult to digest, cause sluggishness of the organs, and clog up the system. Also included in the rajasic category are the spicy, hot, exciting foods that overstimulate the nervous system or sexual glands. All unclean, rotten, and impure food is labeled *tamasic*.

Flesh foods fall into the rajasic category, because they are indeed heavy and difficult to digest. Your body has to work harder and longer to digest meat, especially beef, pork, and lamb, than other foods. For verification, you only have to make the test yourself. Compare how you feel after eating a six-course Chinese dinner, consisting mainly of vegetables and rice, and after a one-course steak dinner. Two hours after you have eaten the Chinese meal, your system will feel light, but after the steak dinner the heavy feeling will still be there.

By and large, this is due to the great amount of cholesterol present in meat. In the last few years the public has been made cholesterol-conscious by unnerving statistics of increasing heart disease and arteriosclerosis. Both these diseases, the layman has been told, are aggravated by cholesterol-rich foods, which are the fatty foods of animal origin. Butter and other animal fats have been declared the enemy, and an alarmed public has learned to cook with polyunsaturated fats and oil. This helped to reduce the intake of cooking fats in the daily diet, but the problem is far from solved, because Americans eat as much meat as they ever did. Most likely, the consistently high amount of meat consumed is the source of the excessive cholesterol in the American diet. Compared to the Europeans who make it a practice to use globs of butter for the rich sauces typical of Continental cooking, Americans do not use much butter; still, we are second only to the Argentineans in our daily consumption of meat. And meat, to the average American, means—except for an occasional lamb chop—beef and pork, the two types of meat containing the most cholesterol. Medical research has shown that Southern blacks, whose diet consists mainly of pork products, suffer the highest degree of hypertension in the United States. Lamb is not quite so high in fat. Next down the list are veal and chicken.

Urging Americans to cut down on meat is almost considered an infringement on the American way of life. I would venture to say that the average American has three meat meals a day—bacon for breakfast, a ham sandwich, hamburger, or hot dog for lunch, and some kind of meat again for dinner. He has been led to believe that meat is necessary to fulfill the daily protein requirement. Yet nutrition studies have revealed that when inhabitants of nations which were affected by meat shortages during World War II were forced to supplement their diet with other protein foods, they were generally healthier than during their meat-eating years. Today, countries where meat consumption is at a minimum report a correspondingly low incidence of the circulatory and rheumatoid diseases so prevalent in this country. We have truly been misled to believe that we must have large quantities of protein to function and that meat is the best source of that protein.

There is as much protein in fish, eggs, and cheese as in

meat, and sometimes even more. Nuts and legumes such as peas, lentils and beans are some of the finest sources of protein. Indeed, there is protein in every living food—in all green leafy vegetables. Yoga considers these last foods the best source of protein and other essential nutrients, because they are the original source. Cattle, lambs, and pigs, the chief suppliers of our meat, get their required protein from vegetables. A steer gets his protein from grass, and we get the protein from the steer. In other words, the protein from meat is strictly secondhand. Some of the vitality in that vegetable life has already been used up by the animal, giving the meat eater a less concentrated amount of food value. The Yogi prefers his protein firsthand, and so passes up meat in favor of foods he considers more beneficial.

Of course, the Yogi who is a vegetarian does not eat only vegetables. He follows an excellent well-rounded diet containing all the essential elements for the body's maintenance and repair—protein, carbohydrates, vitamins, minerals, and fat. He eats all vegetables and fruit, both fresh and dried; nuts; whole wheat grains found in cereals and bread; natural sugar such as honey; and dairy products. A diet like this is the best kind to maintain good health and provide a great amount of energy and stamina.

The Yogi claims that those who become engrossed in Yoga will learn to prefer sattvic foods and forego the rajasic and tamasic foods. This is absolutely true. I personally have undergone a gradual change of likes and dislikes in my daily eating, and all my serious students report the same effect of Yoga on their diets. Heavy and spicy foods interfere with Yoga practice. As you continue in Yoga, you will discover that your appetite will naturally adjust itself, because you will want to eat lightly in order to successfully execute the exercises and to feel well at all times. I have stopped eating meat because I feel better without it, and now have no trouble maintaining my weight. Even the leanest meat is a fattening food in the sense that it is not easily digestible. Although vegetables are the mainstay of my diet, I am not a vegetarian, for I also eat fish and eggs. And in the summertime, when my husband grills steak outdoors, I often succumb to the aroma and have some. As I say, Yoga requires moderation, not deprivation.

Another standard the Yogi uses and which anyone can use to intelligently judge the nutritional value of food is its naturalness. The food eaten in its most natural condition will benefit you the most. Food that has been processed, bleached, refined, and synthesized does considerable harm and has comparatively little food value.

What better place to start applying the standard of naturalness than to bread. Our "staff of life" is the soft, white, packaged variety we buy at the supermarket. To make white bread, the original brown wheat flour must first be bleached, a process that drains it of its natural vitamins and other substances. This procedure originated because people preferred white bread and other white-flour products because of their eye appeal. The miller gladly complied because he discovered that white flour could be stored indefinitely without spoiling. As artificial vitamins became popular, he was able to sell the vitamins he had stripped from the flour to the vitamin manufacturer. Thus, while people are deprived of the natural vitamins and wheat germ contained in whole-wheat flour, they are in the ironic position of buying them back in second- or third-hand concentrations in capsule form. The bread the consumer ended up with was pure starch.

The same bleaching process is applied to other white-flour products, such as noodles, spaghetti, cereal, and cake. They are depleted of their original vitamins and left with virtually nothing but carbohydrates, which are difficult to digest and highly acid-forming. When the lack of nutritional value in white bread and these other products became evident, it was felt necessary to enrich or fortify this food, that is, put in some synthetic vitamins to compensate for the natural vitamins that had been removed. To retard spoilage, food preservatives were often added, some of which are presently under investigation for allegedly containing harmful ingredients.

Like white flour, white polished rice is also pure starch, practically worthless as a nutrient. But brown rice in its natural form is an excellent food. There are also other quite delicious kinds of unpolished rice available from different countries. Try the gourmet shops for these.

Refined sugar is another product that is stripped of its natural food value. The natural sugar cane or sugar beet undergoes many stages of refinement, including the addition of carbon dioxide. I once visited a sugar factory in Barbados, and the stench of the burning sulphur fumes to which the sugar juices were subjected was an unpleasant memory for days. Although devoid of nutrients, these little white granules are powerful stimulants, capable of giving you quick energy, but just as quickly letting you down.

The excess consumption of refined sugar and its products is the prime cause of tooth decay, surely the most prevalent disease in the United States today. To counteract dental cavities, the chemical fluoride has been added to our water, despite warnings from some health authorities that it may damage other parts of the body. A much safer and more direct way to help ensure dental health is to cut down on the intake of refined sugar and the cake, cookies, and candy it is used in.

Refined sugar is an artificial product from a natural food, but sugar substitutes are pure synthetics. Yet as people became calorie-conscious, synthetic sweeteners and synthetically sweetened products became increasingly popular. The harmfulness of saccharin was investigated as early as 1910, and recent studies are turning up strong evidence that artificial sweeteners are a danger to health and certainly should not be used as casually as they are, most likely not at all.

Learn to abandon refined sugar and artificial sweeteners and use honey as a sweetener. If you don't like domestic honey, you'll be surprised to discover the variety of honey from all over the world, which I think is far superior in flavor.

Artificially iodized salt, too, is a synthetic and possesses many harmful qualities when used in excess. Vegetable or sea salt may be substituted for table salt in your cooking. I personally prefer sea salt, which is natural and very gentle. It may cost a few pennies more, but is better-tasting and lends more flavor to your food than table salt.

The combination of salt and nuts is definitely habit-forming. People who start to eat salted nuts can't stop, which is primarily why they are considered fattening. While nuts do contain oil, they are not very fattening when eaten in their natural state—the only way they should be eaten. You cannot always find fresh nuts, but packaged unsalted nuts are usually available. They are a most valuable source of protein. If you're watching your weight, however, don't eat them between meals, as anything additional eaten unnecessarily adds weight. You can introduce them in desserts or as a dessert by themselves.

Whenever you can, serve fresh produce. The availability and convenience of canned and frozen foods, plus the advertising that would have one believe they're as healthful as fresh food, too often lead the housewife to take the lazy way out. So she opens a package or can, serves these lifeless, unappetizing vegetables to her family, and tells her children, "Eat your vegetables; they're good for you." Under the circumstances, we can't blame children for despising vegetables. The extra nutrients you'll be serving your family when you give them fresh food are well worth the extra few minutes and added effort it takes to snap the beans or shell the peas, and the taste of properly cooked fresh vegetables is far superior. Your children will probably be asking for some of these beans and peas raw because they taste so good. In the canning process chemicals are added which, although approved as harmless by the Food and Drug Administration, can't possibly do you any good. Most important in the case for fresh food is the fact that all canned food is precooked and all frozen food preblanched. Any heat treatment of foods causes depletion of nutritional values.

On the whole, the American mother is quite concerned about feeding her family nutritional meals. Her job is not an easy one, especially in the light of all the pressures from her children to buy the artificially flavored, presweetened cereals, candy, and cakes that the television commercials so blatantly tempt them with between the various cartoon shows. Not only that, but she is almost entirely without guidance when it comes to choosing the most nutritious food for her family. Her doctor, unless he's one of the rare ones who have studied nutrition, knows little about it. It wouldn't help to model her meals on the menus planned by most institutions, like schools and hospitals, because these are high in refined and denatured foods. So when she is plagued by doubts that her family is getting the proper food, she tends to cling to the fallacy that she can make up for their nutritional deficiencies by pouring gallons of orange juice and milk into her children and feeding them vitamins. These widely held misconceptions should be examined.

Let's begin with the "gallons of orange juice" fallacy. Of course, oranges are an excellent source of Vitamin C, but so are all citrus fruits, most other fruit, and tomatoes. There are people in countries like Russia and Bulgaria who enjoy great longevity and have never eaten an orange in their lives. One orange eaten whole, preferably with some of the skin, half of a grapefruit, or a tomato adequately fulfills the body's Vitamin

C requirement for the day. And if you've been squeezing your family's orange juice the night before, remember that only orange juice that is drunk immediately after squeezing is high in vitamin content. The longer it is left standing, even refrigerated and covered, the more of its potency is lost. Fresh juice is preferable to canned and frozen juices, which are depleted of their natural vitamins and augmented by artificial Vitamin C.

There are many conflicting theories about milk. Most nutritionists hail the virtues of cow's milk as the ideal food for human beings, yet many children and adults are allergic to it or find it difficult to digest. In most countries of the world, milk drinking is kept to a minimum and goat's milk is considered superior to cow's milk. Others believe that only mother's milk is the proper nourishment for babies. They say only infants should drink milk and the cow's milk was meant for its calf. Take the ancient Greeks who prided themselves on their healthy bodies. They did not drink milk but gave it to their animals instead.

This does not mean that milk is no good. It is an excellent food, high in protein, minerals, and vitamins and easily digestible for the average person. But the same food values are contained in all dairy products. Nor does milk compensate for other vital foods lacking in the diet or for the damage done by too much of the wrong kind of food. Also, most people don't realize that our milk is extremely high in fat content. It compares to the light cream in other countries, while our skim milk is comparable to their regular milk. Anyone with a weight problem, even a small child, should drink skim milk, for it contains the same nutrients, without the added fat content of regular milk.

Finally we come to vitamins. On the whole, we create our own deficiencies by eating the wrong food, then we take artificial vitamins in an effort to alleviate these self-made vitamin deficiencies. Artificial vitamins do have a purpose.

There are times when the body is depleted of vitamins, during or after an illness, during pregnancy and during a metabolic change. Moreover, when fresh foods are not available, artificial vitamins should be taken. But I personally do not believe that artificial vitamins, whether organic or synthetic, should supplement our daily eating. They are a fad and can be dangerous as well as wasteful. Our need for them is a myth created by the vitamin hucksters and supported by so-called nutritionists who make money by writing books and scaring us into thinking that unless we take large amounts of every conceivable vitamin three times a day, terrible diseases will befall us. I know people who have become panicky worrying whether they had their A, B, C, D, E, B+, B_6, B_{12}, iron, phosphorus, magnesium or potassium for the day. The fact is that no one can prescribe exactly how many of this or that vitamin to take, because it is scientifically impossible to determine how much of which vitamins a certain body requires. All vitamins add as they deplete. For instance, if you load up on B_1, you must also take magnesium to counterbalance it, and large doses of C deplete B_{12}. I am not convinced as to the miraculous powers of Vitamin E, and I also do not believe that enormous doses of Vitamin C help prevent the common cold. I believe that it is an unproven and questionable theory, despite the eminence of its advocator, Dr. Linus Pauling, and the testimony of "everybody" who sings its praises. I believe that large doses of anything are harmful to the body. I personally am allergic to Vitamin C, as are many others, and I am convinced that Yoga practice is the answer to common-cold prevention. I do believe in the therapeutic value of vitamin supplements. I have seen tissue restoration in third-degree burn damage, for instance, and I have seen these supplements help victims of severe malnutrition regain their health.

The Yogi also avoids stimulants such as alcohol, coffee, and tea, in addition to heavy and denatured foods. By shocking the nervous system, these beverages, like refined sugar, give you a false feeling of energy that soon ebbs away. It is very easy for an individual to become so addicted to any of these stimulants that he feels he cannot function without it. I am not referring only to excess amounts of alcohol. There are many people who cannot drag themselves out of bed in the morning without first having a cup of coffee, and throughout the day they require frequent refuelings of coffee to keep them going. The side effects of all this caffeine are often insomnia, heartburn, and what has been succinctly termed coffee nerves. As you continue in Yoga, your supply of vitality will increase, and your body will not require these stimulants.

On the other hand, the Yogi does not take a moral stand against coffee, tea, or alcohol. There are Yogis who drink coffee, tea, and wine in moderation. It cannot be denied that there is caffeine in coffee, tannic acid in tea and alcohol in wine, but *moderation* is the key word pertaining to common-sense imbibing. Here are some facts about coffee: Instant or concentrated coffee is subjected to chemical processing and contains harmful additives. Boiled or percolated coffee, especially when left standing, is subjected to the full amount of injurious oils in the coffee bean. Ideally, coffee should be prepared with a filter which absorbs the largest amount of residue and noxious matter, giving you almost pure coffee. Coffee taken black and unsweetened is a food in itself and much less toxic to the system in its undiluted state. Coffee with cream or condensed milk is considered the most harmful combination to the system and the complexion, coffee with milk is milder, and black coffee preferable. I leave it to your good judgment to decide what is best for you.

Who ultimately is responsible for our nutritional standards? Is it the government, the nutritionists, the manufacturers, distributors, advertisers and retailers? Are we the helpless victims of a capitalistic society which has no concern for the individual? Or are we to blame for being lazy, indifferent, unwilling to think for ourselves and ready to shift the blame elsewhere? The answer is obvious, because if we truly realize the importance of proper eating to our general health and are willing to fight for it, we can accomplish substantial changes. There are many angles from which to attack by taking a united stand—the consumer against the government—to change or abolish antiquated nutritional laws and standards. We have already made a big dent in forcing the F.D.A. to halt the spraying of field produce with such harmful repellants as DDT and fluorocarbons, which are deadly to insects and human beings alike. We have been able to effect the ban on proven carcinogenous chemicals, such as Red Dye #2, as additives to food products. We are on the way, at this writing, to force the withdrawal of preservative nitrates and nitrites and to stop the injection of DES to fatten animals—all lethal to human beings. The place to achieve a definite breakthrough in change of eating habits is, of course, in our schools. I am pleased to acknowledge that today in some schools the lunch menus are being revised, and that we are trying to do away with the ghastly foods served in school cafeterias. Canned vegetables and fruits, packaged luncheon meats, white bread, cupcakes, and cookies should eventually be replaced with fresh foods. The PTA must be responsible for these changes and teachers will gladly help. They will teach children to enjoy nutritional foods and to prefer them to junk foods. Cornell University is now doing an extensive study on proper nutrition in the schools, and it is to be hoped that their research will result in healthier eating habits for our young people.

It is almost impossible in this day and age to find food that has not been tampered with in one way or another. But let us not succumb to the dire predictions or scare tactics of some so-called leading nutritionists who would like all foods to be stamped like cigarettes: "Eating Is Dangerous to Your Health." If we are careful about choosing foods and, on the other hand, do not all panic about being poisoned, we can establish a good, healthful way of eating by letting our common sense be the guiding factor.

12

YOGA
AND
EVERYDAY EATING
FOR SLIMNESS

IN OUR MINDS we have come to separate eating for health from eating for pleasure. We tend to turn the first into a burden and the second into guilt. But through Yoga and common sense the two can be combined to include eating for slimness as well.

Yoga has always taught that the slender body is the healthiest body. Today everyone realizes that obesity at any age is a health hazard. It used to be that children had to be fat to be considered healthy. I can still remember the ecstatic cries of appreciation and those mortifying pinches on my fat cheeks from my relatives and my parents' friends at the sight of me as a roly-poly child. Now even the overly fat baby is put on a diet, because an overweight child is more susceptible to sickness than one of normal weight. The modern mother is warned not to gain excessive weight during pregnancy and not to stuff her baby up to the brim, and she is reassured by the pediatrician that it won't die of starvation if it skips a meal. For the middle-aged, obesity is a health risk—and not only in insurance company jargon. In addition to being a health problem, overweight is also a social problem for the teen-ager who is treated like an outcast by his peers, for the unmarried who has difficulty finding a spouse, for the working person in his job. For example, in New York State a schoolteacher or nurse above a prescribed weight cannot be licensed. The myth of the jolly fat person is fast vanishing. Everyone knows it's no fun to be fat.

On the other hand, don't judge your weight by those charts that state what you should weigh at a certain height without taking into account individual body structure. One person may be slim at 135 pounds; another of the same height may be fat. The weight that looks good on one may be unattractive on another. As long as you are firm of flesh, light on your feet, with good health, energy, and stamina, you certainly should not feel like a criminal because statistics label you overweight.

Resist, too, the present popular notion that only the skinny can be attractive and chic. Just as unhealthy as obesity is the other extreme, the trend today toward extreme thinness which becomes an obsession with some women. Regarding any feminine roundness as excess weight, they frantically try to emulate the gaunt models in the high fashion magazines. While the woman with sunken cheeks and a spindly body may be a photogenic mannequin on the printed page, in person she resembles a victim of prolonged starvation— which she probably is. Going along with the prevailing idea that bony means pretty, many young girls with trim, neat figures abandon good sense in an effort to make their body measurements coincide with the spare proportions of their favorite female idols.

Eager to quickly shed unwanted pounds, many people latch on to whatever reducing plan is the current fad. Many of these are potentially as damaging to health as overeating. Some fad diets have caused illness and even death, and those accompanied by diet pills have sometimes led to serious nervous disorders. The medical profession has issued a warning against the so-called fat doctors, who without regard for the patient's health prescribe a variety of reducing drugs, sometimes even indiscriminately over a loudspeaker because they are too busy to see the patient individually.

All fad diets work, because one can lose weight on any monotonous eating routine, whether it's bananas and milk, grapefruit and eggs, all fat foods, all proteins, or steak and wine. They will all produce a weight loss, but the catch is that the effects last for only a short time. As soon as the person returns to his usual eating habits, which is what inevitably happens, the weight reappears, and usually more of it. No pill or extreme diet produces permanent results, because all unhealthful and unnatural forms of eating are rejected by our mental and physical systems in the long run.

All disciplinary eating regimens, such as eating strictly for health or strictly for slimness, lead to frustration if they fail to please the palate. There are some people who are totally uninterested in what they eat and some who are gluttons concerned only with the quantity of food, but the majority of people have strong taste preferences, usually formed in childhood and influenced by advertising. Most people love manufactured sweets and heavy and spicy foods. When they're deprived of these foods, either for reasons of health or weight, they suffer, vocally or silently. Have you ever noticed the martyred expression on the face of a dieter who has just refused a piece of cake? Feeling better physically or wearing a size 10 dress never truly compensates for the loss of eating enjoyment. What commonly happens is that the dieter's feeling of self-pity becomes so overwhelming that he reverts to his old eating habits.

There is, however, a direct approach to a slender figure and good health. It is to develop new tastes in food in order to be able to substitute delicious nonfattening, nutritious food for delicious fattening, unhealthful food. It is quite impossible to learn to enjoy a steady diet of such dull foods as melba toast and plain lettuce leaves, but you can learn to prefer an attractive salad to spaghetti or a delicious piece of fruit cake. You must, of course, forget your food prejudices and keep an open mind. If you say, "But I don't like fish" or "I hate vegetables," it won't work. If you give yourself a chance, you can develop a taste for the foods that are actually best for you.

The only effective reducing plan I know of for someone who has to lose a lot of weight, say fifty or a hundred pounds, is offered by the diet clubs which in recent years have sprung up all over the country. They have various names but follow the basic principles of Alcoholics Anonymous. The clubs have centers where people meet—men, women, or children who are all in the same overweight boat—and frankly discuss their individual problems, which become easier to handle as mutual problems. The idea is to lose weight through eating rather than starvation, to fill up on low-calorie food so there is little craving for high-calorie food. Medicines to stimulate weight loss are taboo. The members follow the simple commonsense diet published by the Department of Health. The diet may not be ideal from the Yogic point of view, but it is certainly much healthier than all fad diets. It is a reducing plan that can keep the pounds off. After the initial weight loss, the new style of eating can be maintained, because it is satisfying and appealing.

All her life Mother claimed she had heavy bones and therefore couldn't lose weight. At my urging, she joined one of these diet clubs and, heavy bones to the contrary, took off thirty pounds. That was five years ago, but she has kept it off. After her initial weight loss, she was less strict with herself, but her new eating habits prevail. At eighty, she looks and feels great.

Good eating habits are an insurance policy for a healthy and good-looking old age. If they are established in childhood, so much the better, but like Yoga they prove beneficial at any stage of life. Healthful eating of fresh, life-giving foods will not only prevent internal deterioration but external deterioration as well. The dreadful meals consumed by American youth, consisting largely of soda pop, hot dogs, hamburgers, pizzas, French fries, potato chips, white bread, cake, and candy at first seem to have had no evident physical effects, but studies of Viet Nam war victims have shown that soldiers as young as twenty often were in poor cardiovascular health, at the onset or in the advanced stages of atherosclerosis, arthritis, diabetes, etc. While our young people are outwardly pictures of health, with good skin and teeth and rosy cheeks, the senior citizen and the average middle-aged American tend toward sagging skin, unhealthy palates, varicose veins, liver spots, sunken eyes, false teeth, and hair loss. We have greater access to camouflage and repair than anyone else in the world—to cosmetics, creams, toupees, girdles, and face lifts—but there are always mirrors to be faced. Let's not forget paunches and spare tires and superfluous fat anywhere. Statistics have proven that slimness in old age is one of the most important factors in warding off disease, and that weight stability is an essential factor in establishing well-being. Proper exercising, an optimistic outlook, meaningful productivity, and a healthy environment all play an important part in retaining good health and good looks in old age, but good nutrition is the key to a youthful appearance. Yogis in their eighties are wrinkle-free, most likely have their own teeth, and usually have abundant hair growth and thin, sinewy bodies. Studies of the Hunza people in the Northwest range of the Himalayas have proven that diet is the main factor in their unusual health and longevity.

Once you have accustomed your body to a proper diet, it will prefer the light nutritional foods and you will have no problem rejecting other kinds of food. Through the Yoga exercises and principles of nutrition, you are reeducating your body to know what is best for you. Most people, especially those over forty, are ten or fifteen pounds overweight. When you do the Yoga exercises your body will start complaining about this excess baggage, for these few extra pounds will interfere with the execution of the exercises. With the combination of physical activity and a change in eating habits, it will not be difficult to lose that weight.

Keep in mind that drastic weight fluctuation is harmful to the system, especially in and past middle age. A sudden loss of weight is likely to cause sagging and wrinkling of your face and body. Weight loss should not exceed a pound a week. (This excludes the drastically overweight.) Ideally, weight should come off at the rate of two pounds a month. This is the only way it stays off, and you keep looking well.

Whenever someone speaks of a weight problem, it is immediately assumed the problem is overweight. But being underweight is also a problem. It is really more difficult to gain weight than to lose it. However, there is little compassion for the underweight. When they complain that nothing they eat adds pounds, they usually meet with an unsympathetic response, like "I should have your problems!" The solution is not to stuff oneself with sugars, starches, and fats, for an excess of these foods will do as much damage to an underweight person as to anyone else. The problem can usually be traced to metabolism and nerves. Performing the Yoga exercises will help release tension and stimulate the glands, so the body can effectively utilize the food that is consumed. Supplied with the proper diet, the body will build itself up and maintain its correct weight.

Healthful eating, in the broadest sense of the term, is not only *what* you eat but *how* you eat. In addition to being a basic drive, eating should constitute one of our greatest pleasures. A meal should represent a break in our routine, an enjoyable interlude spent with family or friends or alone, and a treat to the senses. It should not be regarded as a mere necessity, a time to fill the stomach as you fill the gas tank of your car, a hurried affair to be got over as quickly as possible.

Some predict that one of the marvels the world of the future has in store for us is that all food will come in the form of pills. Presumably breakfast, lunch, and dinner will then be no more than three quick swallows. Certainly the trend seems to be moving in that direction, with all the instant and concentrated food crowding the supermarket shelves. We can do our bit to forestall this appalling prospect by personally reviving good eating and good eating habits.

Eating tuna fish out of the can may make you less hungry, but an appetizing salad will be more satisfying. In the average household, the dining room, tablecloth, and good dishes are reserved strictly for company. I'm not suggesting that you use these every day, but do pay more attention to the surroundings of daily meals. Even a kitchen table can be set attractively with place mats and nice dishes. Any picture is enhanced by an attractive frame, and the simplest food will be more appetizing when served attractively.

Take time for meals. Granted, this is a tall order to fill for the harassed housewife with babies clinging all over her, but one that will benefit her and her family more than she realizes. Set aside time for a leisurely dinner, either alone with your husband or with him and the older children. Try to choose a time that is convenient for all, and insist they be on time. This can be one of the most enjoyable times of the day for everyone, not just an annoying interruption in a television program. The mother, to whom dinnertime can come to be only a burdensome chore of preparing, serving, and cleaning up afterwards, should try to relax as well and enjoy both her food and her family. Difficult as that may seem, consider it a necessity to help fight the increasing tensions that we are all subjected to.

One of the gospels of Yoga is that to masticate properly is the answer to most digestive troubles. The healthy stomach of the normal person can cope with almost any food if that food has been thoroughly chewed. On the other hand, even the most nutritional food that has not been completely chewed often cannot be effectively used by the body. The digestive process begins in the mouth, where the digestive juices go to work breaking down the food so it can be absorbed by the body as nourishment. If the food particles are too large they cannot be easily digested and may pass out the large intestine without having been utilized by the body.

Thorough chewing is also a great weapon against obesity. Those who chew slowly can truly taste and enjoy the food that they are eating, instead of finishing quickly and craving the next course. Just as good wine should be sipped and savored, so should each morsel of food. When this is done, the stomach will be satisfied before it is satiated and will let you know when it has had enough.

Chewing is also healthy exercise for the gums and teeth. Children should be given carrots and bread crusts to chew on instead of chewing gum, which should be eliminated because of its harmful effects on teeth.

Another Yoga principle that makes very good sense is to eat only when you are hungry. Some people can go all day without food and require only one large meal. Others must eat more often in smaller quantity. Eat as your stomach, not the clock, commands. It is good and natural to feel hunger. A healthy appetite means not the capacity to devour great quantities of food, but the ability to enjoy food when one is hungry.

There is no reason to stick to a three-meals-a-day routine if you feel more comfortable eating only two. It was the custom of the health-conscious ancient Greeks to eat just two meals. Many families have got into the Sunday brunch habit, combining breakfast and lunch around eleven or twelve and then having a light dinner in the evening. They find the two meals quite adequate for the day.

Eating a large meal at noon and a light meal in the evening is healthier than eating the large meal at the end of the day. However, since this is not feasible for most people because of their work schedule, it is best to eat as early as possible, to avoid going to bed with a full stomach, a common cause of indigestion, constipation, and overweight.

Avoid eating when you are tense and overtired. At these times, when the whole organism is affected adversely, food taken in is apt to do more harm than good.

If you are a meat eater, try to cut down on your meat intake. Substitute poultry for red meat whenever possible, and completely forget about hot dogs, sausages, bacon, ham, and all other smoked meats, for most of them contain nitrates, nitrites, and other chemicals; and if you saw or smelled the inferior quality of the leftover meats that go into sausage, you would never again subject your body to such outrage.

Avoid all manufactured or packaged foods with the few exceptions of beans, dried peas, lentils, all other legumes, whole wheat cereal and brown rice. To play it safe, forego any packaged foods that list among their contents any additives in one form or other to insure freshness, prevent spoilage, insure long shelf life, add color, or promote palatability. All additives are synthetic, and most are harmful. All packaged, frozen, canned, pickled, and smoked foods are denatured, devoid of natural vitamins, and harmful. All canned and bottled soft drinks should also be avoided. They all contain sugar or worse—artificial sweeteners—and they are unhealthful.

Yoga advises that as one grows older, especially after thirty-five, one should eat less to maintain perfect health. It stands to reason that the body that is no longer growing but only carrying on maintenance and repair work does not need so much food. Also, most people lead less physically active lives as they get older and do not burn up so many calories as they did when they were younger. The surplus turns into a burden of fat for the body to carry around.

The same advice about overeating holds true for overdrinking. Water is the most healthful drink of all, but the generally accepted rule about drinking eight glasses of water a day is without foundation. Unless you are under doctor's orders to drink a prescribed amount of water daily, you should let your own body prescribe the amount of water best for you. Drink when you are thirsty, not to fulfill some arbitrary quota. Plain tap water is fine; well water is better. If you are not fortunate enough to be supplied with it in your area, make an effort to buy it bottled. It does not cost very much.

The habit of drinking iced water or any iced beverage is an unhealthy one. Ice produces a shock when it comes in contact with the skin. Imagine, then, what a jolt it can cause to your digestive and nervous systems.

Generally speaking, it is not a good idea to drink with meals. Drinking while eating tends to result in overeating and washing food down instead of thoroughly chewing it. However, once you have established your suitable weight, you could adopt the good habit of having a glass of dry wine with dinner. It adds a festive touch to any meal and is low in calories. Since it is sipped, not poured down, it is an aid to digestion. A glass of good wine before supper can also take the place of a high-calorie cocktail.

Raw juices are a wonderful health booster. Their benefits could prove valuable to your health and that of your family. It is a time-consuming process to prepare and squeeze vegetables and fruits, and most of their juices have to be drunk immediately for maximum food value. Also, a vegetable juicer is an expensive appliance. On the other hand, let me assure those who feel they must supplement their diets with artificial vitamins that both monetarily and healthwise, a juicer is in the long run cheaper and a superior investment. Freshly squeezed vegetable and fruit juices are of great therapeutic value to sufferers from many chronic ailments. In their concentrated form, raw juices are the most regenerating food for building and maintaining good health. Carrot juice, especially, one of the richest sources of Vitamin A, is frequently called a miracle juice for the cure and prevention of numerous ailments. Regular drinking of carrot juice can stop chronic colds, help curb chronic kidney and bladder diseases, and strengthen the eyes.

The enthusiasm for raw juices shouldn't be carried to extremes, however. I know someone who drank carrot juice to the exclusion of everything else and became a victim of carotene poisoning.

Yoga recommends periodic fasts to cleanse the body and rest the digestive organs, which are otherwise constantly working. You should especially make it a point to fast during sickness. You will note that animals do not eat when they are sick. This is nature's safeguard while the body is working to regain health. During your fast you may drink water, water with lemon, vegetable juice, or vegetable broth when you get hungry. You may feel hungry at first, but your hunger pangs will subside. If you can, go through the night without eating, but if you are too uncomfortable by evening, eat a light meal—a vegetable, baked potato, and beverage, unsweetened and without milk. For those with digestive trouble, an enema the night before fasting is usually advised.

Fasting, incidentally, is the most effective way of reducing. If you are on a low-calorie, three-meals-a-day diet, for instance, you will find yourself suffering feelings of hunger from one skinny meal to the next. If you stop eating completely, you will experience hunger pains for only one day.

The next day you will feel great and on the ensuing days greater, and the fat will roll off. Drink only when thirsty and avoid coffee, tea, and all toxins. You can work and exercise and you will not feel weak. The more weight you have to lose, the longer you can keep fasting. Remember, though, that no prolonged fast should be undertaken without medical supervision.

Before going into some particulars of sensible, healthy everyday diets, I'd like to direct a few words to the housewife who is in charge of it all. The responsibility for your family's nutrition is yours. It is up to you to decide which foods are good and which are not. Don't throw your family into a panic by suddenly depriving them of all the foods they are used to, but gradually substitute good food for bad food. Buy the best food in season and prepare it attractively.

Most people hold the mistaken opinion that simple, natural cooking and eating is dull. Nothing is further from the truth. By nature and avocation I am a gourmet who loves good food and loves to cook. I can spend hours browsing in gourmet shops. I find some of my most exciting reading in cookbooks and can turn out a hollandaise sauce or a soufflé with the best of them, but I seldom do, for I have completely changed my style of cooking. Whereas I used to prepare food in the heavily sauced Continental manner, I now cook with regard to naturalness, lightness, and healthfulness, but with no less attention to taste and flavor.

By using herbs and exotic spices, you'll discover a whole new world of flavor without having to add butter and cream to enhance the natural taste of food. Try any of these: dill, parsley, chervil, chives, sage, marjoram, caraway seeds, thyme, paprika, garlic, onions, leeks, rosemary, oregano, cumin seed or powder, turmeric, and curry in moderation. For extra flavoring, try the concentrated seasoning cubes available in health-food stores.

A word about cooking methods. Food should be boiled,

broiled, or baked. Although no food should be deep fried, occasionally it may be sautéed, which means fried lightly, preferably in the specially coated pans that require very little shortening. Use vegetable oil or a little butter for cooking. While margarine may be slightly lower in cholesterol, it is a synthetic food.

The number one rule to remember when preparing vegetables is never to overcook them. Either steam or pressure-cook them, or use a pot with a heavy bottom. Barely cover the vegetables with water, bring them quickly to a boil, lower the flame, and simmer carefully only until tender. You can reserve the cooking water for soup base.

Following the menu suggestions below are some recipes that the Yoga student could use for tasty and healthy eating. I have given special consideration to weight watchers. Bear in mind that these menus mention only a few of the possibilities available. They're intended not as a complete list but only to spark your imagination.

Breakfast

Right now, first thing in the morning, is the time to begin relying on the judgment of your own body and mind, instead of what people tell you. Forget that you "must" have a big breakfast. You must never eat when you're not hungry or force your children to do so. Some people enjoy a hearty meal early in the morning; others shudder at the thought of it. If you don't feel like having breakfast, drink a glass of water or some other beverage, or have a piece of fruit.

If you are hungry, there is a large variety of food to choose from. If you want juice, make it freshly squeezed, or as an alternative, you can use the juice that comes in glass jars without sugar or sweetener added. Any fresh fruit is excellent; oranges, grapefruit, bananas or apples in the winter and melons, berries, or peaches in the summer—to name but a few.

For cold cereal, find a whole wheat, unsweetened one, and avoid the boxes which list mysterious abbreviations that stand for harmful chemicals. Eat it with skim milk, sliced fruit, and honey. Add a generous tablespoon of wheat germ. Be on the lookout for imported packaged cereals that contain wheat germ, wheat and millet flakes, organically grown fruit, and no storage preservatives. For hot cereal, stick to oatmeal with skim milk, honey, fruit, and wheat germ, or if you have no weight problem, cream of wheat or cream of rice.

You could make some pancakes from wheat flour, of course. Or have an egg once in a while—one. Limit your intake of eggs to four to six per week. With it have a slice of bread or toast, whole wheat or rye, but not with butter or margarine. On your bread try cottage cheese, with honey or apple butter to satisfy that craving for something sweet.

Have your beverage.

Lunch

If you ate a large breakfast, go easy on lunch. If you can skip it, do so by all means, but never at the expense of being ravenous by suppertime. If you have to eat twice as much at dinner because you've gone without lunch, you are doubly defeating your purpose. Maybe you can get by comfortably on just a snack. Try yogurt. It can easily be taken with you and eaten anywhere. It would be best to eat it plain or with honey, but if you like it with the preserves added to commercial yogurt, don't worry too much about those relatively few calories. If you have the time and initiative, you can make your own yogurt, which is superior to the store-bought varieties. Yogurt is sometimes regarded almost as some sort of magic elixir. It is not; it is simply a fine food because it is nutritious, filling, easily digestible, and low in calories.

Cottage cheese is another food you should get acquainted with. Living in a competitive country, you have many brands from which to choose, some tastier than others. Farmer cheese, pot cheese and ricotta are also excellent foods, filling and easy to digest. Spices and herbs can be added for extra flavor. Next come the hard cheeses such as Swiss or American, but keep away from the rich, soft, fermented, or heavily spiced cheeses.

Try to limit your daily intake of bread to two slices. If you had bread for breakfast, omit the usual sandwich. Lunch does become somewhat of a problem for the worker or schoolchild who has to bring his lunch, but with ingenuity an alternative to the sandwich can be found: a piece of cold chicken or fish with raw vegetables or a fresh fruit or cottage-cheese salad with wheat crackers. If you must have a sandwich, make a sincere effort to get away from sausage, ham, and all meat. Also, go easy on canned fish. Eliminate mayonnaise, catsup, and prepared mustard, three unhealthy condiments. You could eat your single egg for lunch, hardboiled, with lettuce and tomato in a sandwich. Another choice would be some kind of cheese sandwich, even cream cheese, unless you are overweight. The same goes for peanut butter, which is an excellent food when not accompanied by the standard jelly and white bread. Even the weight watchers should try an avocado sandwich. The avocado contains almost every nutrient needed by the system. One could live exclusively on avocados and enjoy excellent health.

Have a beverage *after* the meal.

Supper or Dinner

It is a good idea, especially for the weight watcher, to have a beverage a half-hour before dinner: fresh vegetable juice, vegetable broth, or skim milk. Any of these will diminish your initial hunger and enable you to start dinner in a leisurely manner instead of greedily.

Start dinner with fresh fruit, such as grapefruit or melon. They are your best dietetic friends, low in calories.

Or begin dinner with soup. As a labor of love, make your family homemade soup. Soup is not fattening unless you add butter and cream, unnecessary embellishments to vegetable, pea, bean, or lentil soup.

Learn to substitute fish for meat. Many people don't like fish because they have not been educated toward it from childhood, but a taste for it can be developed. Find a good fish store with a reputation for fresh fish. No doubt you will be surprised at the variety of fish available besides the familiar old stand-bys you're used to. Keep an open mind about trying new kinds. Your fish man can advise you what to buy and how to prepare it. He will also bone and fillet it for you.

All fish or seafood is high in vitamins and minerals and easily digestible. It can be broiled, baked, or sautéed. Do not eat smoked fish, such as salmon, because it is loaded with nitrite. Canned fish, such as tuna and salmon, has no nutritional value whatsoever, and shellfish or anything that swims near the shore is affected by polluted waters. Try to choose a deep-ocean fish. It can also contain traces of mercury, but chances of this are slim. Fish from mountain rivers and streams is also very edible.

The meats that are most overlooked in this country are the relatively inexpensive organ meats. The only one with some degree of popularity is liver, an excellent source of protein and abundant vitamins, to be sure. But there are others equally good, healthy, and easy to digest: kidneys, brains, sweetbreads, tripe, and lungs.

Chicken, whether baked, broiled, or boiled, is not so valuable a food as fish or the organ meats, but is easily digestible and may be included in a good diet. Turkey and duck belong in the heavy-food category.

Have a salad and one or two cooked vegetables with your fish or meat. Get acquainted with all the varieties of lettuce and other salad plants there are—Boston, bibb, romaine, chicory, etc. Iceberg lettuce seems to be the most popular but is lowest in vitamin content. Anything green and fresh may be used in a salad, even those we usually cook, such as spinach, cabbage, and turnip greens. If you are in doubt as to whether to cook it, don't. Cut, dice, or break it into a salad instead, along with tomatoes, radishes, cucumbers, red and green peppers, watercress, and avocado. Red and white onions, scallions, parsley, and dill do wonders for a salad.

Use vegetable oil in your salads instead of olive oil. It is lighter and lower in calories and—combined with salt, pepper, and herbs—quite tasty. Your dressing can be made with oil and lemon, or if you like, you may use a little good-quality vinegar instead of the lemon juice. Fresh lemon juice, by the way, should be used liberally on all raw and cooked food.

Most people get into a rut with vegetables, serving the same ones continually, never taking full advantage of the variety offered. Experiment with the herbs listed earlier in this chapter. They lend added interest to vegetables. To get back to those fresh string beans: cook them for seven minutes in a minimum amount of salted water, drain, and add a little butter, dill, and seasoning. You will never revert to the canned or frozen kind.

Potatoes and brown and unpolished rice are valuable foods and should not be neglected, even by the dieter. You may have a rice dish, a nonstarchy vegetable and a salad or a baked potato. And try cottage cheese and chives on your baked potato next time. Rice or potato with yogurt is a nice combination too.

Fruit is the best solution to the problem of desserts. Take advantage of fruits in season and eat as much as you like of them. A fresh fruit salad with honey, berries in season, and fresh pineapple in winter are a few successful substitutes for gooey desserts. For those with no weight problem, there is custard or pudding, made with honey instead of sugar. There are also nuts and dried fruit, raisins, dates, figs, apricots, apples, and plums to appease a sweet tooth. They are excellent snacks for children, too, instead of other sweets. The natural sugar they contain will produce natural energy without promoting tooth decay or aggravating disease. Yes, they're fattening, but not so much so as cake, cookies, and candy.

Have your beverage after your meal.

Here are some of my favorite recipes from all over the world. I haven't always given exact measurements for seasoning, because I season according to my taste and advise you to do the same.

Accompanied by a salad, either of these two soup dishes is a meal in itself.

FISH SOUP (from Spain)

2 pounds fish (mackerel, bass, whitefish, bluefish, pike, etc.), cut into serving pieces
2 pounds seafood (mussels, clams, shrimp, crabs, scallops, etc.)
1 cup chopped onion
½ cup chopped Italian parsley
2 cups chopped tomatoes
1 clove garlic, minced
1 cup dry white wine
2 cups water
1/3 cup vegetable oil

Heat a large kettle, and add the oil. Sauté onion and garlic until light brown, then add the parsley and tomatoes. Season well with salt, freshly ground pepper, and oregano. Cook over medium flame for 10 minutes. Pour in water and wine and bring to a boil. Add the fish and seafood, except for the mussels and clams. Simmer for 20 minutes. Add mussels and clams, and simmer until they open. Add more water if needed.

CHICKEN IN THE POT (International)

3- to 4-pound chicken, quartered
2 pounds beef bones
2 onions
4 ribs celery
A few sprigs parsley
Thyme, if available
Seasoning cubes and salt, as desired
6 peeled carrots
Other vegetables suggested: small cabbage, quartered; small cauliflower, quartered; Brussels sprouts; small potatoes

Cover all the ingredients with water in a large kettle except carrots and the other suggested vegetables. Season, and bring to a boil. Cover, and simmer for 45 minutes. Discard bones, onions, celery, and parsley. Add all the other vegetables. Cook for another 20 minutes or until everything is tender. Sprinkle with fresh parsley before serving.

Here are two party dips, not exactly without calories but not loaded with them either, and extremely nutritious. If you can find it, warm pitah, a flat Eastern bread, is very good eaten with these dips.

HUMUS *(Middle East)*

1-pound package chickpeas
1 teaspoon garlic juice or garlic powder
Juice of ½ lemon
½ cup vegetable oil
Salt, freshly ground pepper to taste
Finely chopped parsley

Soak chickpeas overnight. Discard water. Cover with fresh water, add a little salt, and cook until very soft, about 45 minutes. Drain, and mix peas and other ingredients into a smooth paste in an electric blender. Add more oil or a little water, if needed. Serve cold, sprinkled with parsley.

GUACAMOLE *(Mexican)*

1 large, very ripe avocado
Juice of 1 lemon
Salt, pepper, garlic, Worcestershire sauce to taste
1 small onion, grated
½ cup combined cream cheese and sour cream or, for weight watchers, ½ cup cottage cheese and yogurt

Mash avocado with fork to a smooth consistency with no lumps. Add other ingredients and mix until creamy but not watery. Chill.

Helpful hint: Leave the avocado pit in the guacamole until serving time, to prevent the mixture from turning dark.

SABRA SALAD *(Israel)*

1 avocado, cut into chunks
2 cucumbers, peeled and cut up
2 large tomatoes, cut up
1 fresh green or red pepper, cut up
Bunch of radishes, sliced

Bunch of scallions (use the green tops also), chopped
Vegetable oil, salt, and freshly ground pepper

Add all ingredients in a large bowl, mix, and chill well.

MY FAVORITE COLE SLAW

1 firm head of cabbage
1 tablespoon caraway seeds
1 tablespoon imported mustard
Juice of 2 lemons, or 1/3 cup vinegar
1/3 cup oil
Salt, pepper, and a dash of sugar

Cut cabbage very fine. Add all ingredients and mix well. For variation add grated apple, grated onion, diced fresh red or green peppers.

SQUASH FILLED WITH MUSHROOMS

1 large acorn squash
½ pound fresh mushrooms
½ cup diced onion
Butter and seasoning

Cut squash in half, remove seeds, add a dab of butter to the cavity and bake in 350° oven for 30 minutes. Heat oil in pan, sauté onion and sliver-sliced mushrooms with salt and pepper until browned. Fill the squash with the mixture, top with bread crumbs and dabs of butter. Put under broiler for five minutes and serve.

FILLET OF SOLE A LA INA

Put the fillets of sole into a bowl with some seasonings, salt, and black pepper, and let stand for a half-hour. Then turn the fish over a couple of times in a mixture of Parmesan cheese and bread crumbs. Fry in buttered pan five to six minutes on each side. At the same time, fry mushrooms and parsley in a little butter in another pan and pour the mixture over the fish just before serving.

STRAWBERRY DELIGHT

1 cup yogurt
2 cups cottage cheese
2 teaspoons honey
1/3 cup orange juice
1 teaspoon vanilla
Strawberries

Combine all ingredients except the strawberries in a blender and whip until fluffy. Serve over strawberries. Absolutely delicious!

A Yogi friend who is the acclaimed gourmet in Yoga circles gave me these two Indian recipes. I omit the potent chili peppers and chili and curry powders characteristic of Indian cooking.

RICE WITH NUTS AND RAISINS

1 cup Indian rice, washed well
½ cup natural pistachio or pine nuts
½ cup raisins
1 tablespoon butter or ghee (clarified butter)
4 cups water
Salt, turmeric, cumin seed, and mustard seed

Put rice, water, salt, nuts, and raisins in a pot. Bring to a boil, with the pot uncovered, and continue boiling for 15 minutes. Keep testing the rice with a fork for doneness. Roll one grain between your fingers to be sure it is perfectly cooked. Do not overcook. Drain the excess water from the rice with a colander. Melt the butter in the hot pot with the flame off, stir in the spices, and add the rice. Stir well and cover. Do not heat again.

EGGPLANT AND BANANAS

1 medium eggplant
2 ripe bananas, unpeeled, washed well
1 large tomato, chopped
1 large green or red pepper, chopped
½ cup vegetable oil
Salt, pepper, turmeric, cumin seed, and mustard seed

Bake eggplant in 350° oven for about 30 minutes. If the skin is tender, leave it on; if you are in doubt, peel off the skin. Heat the oil in a heavy casserole, and add spices. Slice the bananas thickly and sauté for about 10 minutes. Add the tomato and pepper and cook for 10 more minutes. Cut the eggplant into chunks and add to the casserole. Stir lightly and cook another 5 minutes or until tender. Do not overcook.

In conclusion, don't think that you must renounce forever certain foods that you and your family consider delicious, simply because they don't come up to Yoga standards of eating. However, learn to reserve them for occasional treats. Don't feel guilty about having a good piece of chocolate, a rich cake, or a martini. Enjoy them once in a while, but not as a steady diet. As you begin to appreciate the vital natural foods, the rich foods will lose their appeal. You'll be eating healthier food and enjoying it more.

13

YOGA
AND
YOU

IF YOU'RE STILL WONDERING whether Yoga is what you are looking for, I say give it a try.

By now you've probably tried all the other physical exercise
programs and entered into all of them with great enthusiasm.
Perhaps you became a member of a health club, intrigued by
all the gadgets that would firm and slim you effortlessly, or
even invested in a mechanical exercising gadget of your own.
Or if you were energetic, you attended calisthenics classes,
exercised to television, followed the instructions of various
books, or jogged along faithfully in rain or shine, oblivious to
curious stares and adept at dodging traffic. You pursued these
activities faithfully, and they did you a world of good. You felt
better, looked better, and became trimmer and firmer. But that

inevitable day came when your enthusiasm began to ebb, then disappeared completely. You just couldn't stand the thought of another push-up, isometric, or ride on the exercycle, and you stopped. If you think your case is unique, be assured it's not. Just glance through the classified ads in the Sunday newspaper offering used gym equipment for sale, sometimes to be had for the hauling.

Don't berate yourself for lack of willpower, for most physical self-improvement plans are doomed to failure. No one is going to voluntarily keep doing something he doesn't like. Furthermore, when you have to force yourself to do something because it may be good for you, you are defeating your purpose, because the tensions you bring to a task you dislike are harmful to your body. Like the steady diet of lettuce leaves and melba toast mentioned earlier, a steady diet of these kinds of physical exercises is just no fun. Hatha Yoga is different. That is why Yoga is superior to other forms of exercise. For the moment I'm not even considering its added advantages of breathing techniques and mental benefits. Yoga will do you more good and you'll want to practice, because Yoga is *fun* to do.

You will look forward to exercising, and once you have established it as part of your routine, you won't want to give it up. If you should skip the exercises, your body will let you know that it is missing something vital to its well-being. Yoga will become part of you, giving you lasting benefits all your life.

People generally believe that they are physically fit because they play tennis, jog, bicycle, or swim. The Sunday golfer is fooling himself into believing that his eighteen holes are a decisive factor in maintaining good health. Many Americans think that sports are the answer to physical exercise, but sports are really more of a diversion for leisure time and cannot provide you with overall physical fitness. Sports are fun and good for your figure, health and morale, but there is no one sport that conditions your whole body. Athletes in general are in pretty bad shape, prone to backaches, other muscular aches, pulls, sprains, dislocated vertabrae and discs. One reason for this is that in their particular sport or event they concentrate on developing only certain parts of their anatomy, often subjecting these to continuous stress. If you indulge in one sport exclusively, while ignoring the body structure as a whole, you can severely damage yourself. Baseball, tennis, and horseback riding, for example, demand extreme forward movement of the muscles. Unless the muscles are also worked in the reverse direction, the body is subject to charley horse, extreme stiffness, muscular strain, and tension.

Most sports, such as football, baseball, tennis, swimming, bicycling, and jogging, tend to shorten the very muscles that are necessary for participation in the sport. Examples of this are the tightening of the hamstrings, in playing ball; chronic injuries to the Achilles tendon, in running; tennis elbow; football knee; and general inflammation and irritation of muscles and joints. In competitive sports, the tension, anxiety, and stress that build up before the event invariably result in muscle tightness and present the most prevalent cause of injury in any sport.

Perfect physical condition is attained when every area of the body is exercised and every muscle is reached. There must be consistent convex, concave, and lateral movement to achieve superb flexibility of the spine, the legs, and the whole body.

Yoga can help you do better in any sport. I have worked with tennis players and horseback riders who found that Yoga lessened all the symptoms caused by jerky forward movement and conditioned their bodies to withstand the specific stresses of those sports. Tennis players can improve their endurance and grip and can prevent tennis elbow or work it out through Yoga. Swimmers have reported their increased breath control and endurance, and skiers and skaters have noticed improvement of coordination. Yoga training decreases their chance of getting hurt when they fall, because they learn to have better control of their bodies. Yoga develops powerful abdominal muscles, and those who participate in martial arts find it extremely helpful.

Years ago the champion French Olympic Ski Team used Yoga as part of its training, though it is only lately that American sports teams are incorporating Yoga conditioning exercises into their preparations for the actual sport. Many trainers of football, baseball, and hockey teams have recognized that the way to avoid injuries caused by the foreshortening and tightening of the musculature is to stretch, loosen, elongate, and elasticize the muscles beforehand, and that Yoga is the perfect conditioner. They have recognized that a relaxed body will stay free from injury and that a relaxed mind can withstand the tension and strain of competition. The body and mind control, the concentration and coordination learned through Yoga exercise and breathing make for better athletes. We see pictures of individual athletes in Yoga practice—Mark Spitz, Olympic swimmer; Jean-Claude Killy, Olympic skier; Chris Evert, tennis champion; and Bob Snyder, pitcher for the Baltimore Orioles.

Yoga does require self-discipline. I purposely use the term self-discipline instead of willpower because willpower implies forcing yourself to do something against your nature, whereas self-discipline is simply fulfilling an obligation to yourself. The benefits that Yoga offers are attractive, but you have to work to achieve them. In the beginning, you'll have to give yourself the little push to set aside the time to practice when you think you're too tired, and to keep at it. After a short time the momentum of Yoga will take over, and you'll find you won't need to give yourself that push, for Yoga will have become a part of you.

Don't confuse push with rush. Don't start Yoga with the idea of accomplishing as much as you possibly can in the shortest span of time. The eager beaver who wants to learn everything immediately and throws himself into a frenzy of practice in the beginning never sticks with Yoga very long— or, for that matter, with anything he begins, but is forever rushing into something new.

There are other don'ts to remember in Yoga. Don't become impatient with your body if at first it seems resistant to your wishes. The back that won't straighten or the knees that won't bend will respond sooner and better to gentle prodding than to brute force. Your body will learn to assume the positions, but it is a gradual process. The stiffness has been acquired over years. You'll regain resiliency, and it won't take years. In fact, it will take a relatively short time, but everything can't be accomplished overnight. You could hurt yourself if your impatience forces your body into a position it's not yet ready to assume.

Don't set your goals too high, especially in the beginning. Don't aim for acrobatic feats that others may be executing with what appears to be effortless ease. While you should be aware of your present capacity, you should not make up your mind that a certain pose is impossible. Concentrate on perfecting each pose to the best of your ability. When one of my students tells me, "I can't do this now, but someday I will," he has grasped the meaning of Yoga and is well on his way to success.

No one is born to success. Anything worth achieving requires diligence and very often purely mechanical practice. A person may be born with a natural talent for singing, dancing, or painting, but unless he works to develop that talent, it will amount to nothing. The daily repetition of scales, pliés, or brush strokes is necessary to make a great artist, and it is consistency that brings the desired results. The same is true for Yoga. You will find Yoga practice quite rewarding, because your body will respond quickly.

For the best results in Yoga, find a teacher. It is possible to learn Yoga by the book, just as it's possible to become a lawyer by a correspondence course, but it's not the best way. In classic Yoga literature, it is advised that you seek a Guru of infinite wisdom, at whose lotus feet you should worship, one who will be your mother, father, and master, and who will lead you to physical and mental perfection. Although there are dissatisfied persons all over the world desperately seeking to follow such a Guru, I would advise you not to expect all that from any teacher. A good teacher can become a friend to turn to for advice, but certainly shouldn't be worshiped.

Although some individual teachers hand out Teacher's Training Certificates after completion of a course, they have no validity. Unfortunately no official licensing for Yoga teachers exists to date, which is why anyone can call himself a Yoga teacher. I know of many teachers who have learned Yoga from TV or from a book and have never taken a lesson. There are calisthenics and dance teachers who slow down their movement and call this Yoga because it is more lucrative.

Use your common sense: inquire into a teacher's background. Where did he get his training? How long has he taught? What are his qualifications?

Let me give you my definition of a good Yoga teacher, and the qualifications that I require from my teachers. He or she must look good, and I don't mean a beautiful face or perfect figure, but a healthy appearance, good posture, and no flabbiness anywhere. (Otherwise you can be assured that they do not practice what they teach.) A pleasing voice and a pleasant and unhurried way of speaking are necessities. A good

teacher does not exercise along with the class. He demon-
strates the posture and then moves around the room to direct
and assist. He must know when and how to touch (or not
touch) the student's body to help him reach certain positions.
All my teachers are knowledgeable in anatomy and kinesiology, either through professional backgrounds or by going to
school for these subjects. My teachers love Yoga and devote
part of their time to improving their own techniques. They
have a genuine desire to help people and are willing to impart
their store of energy to their students. They are warm and
outgoing. All my teachers start as beginner students with me,
and when I recognize their potential as Yoga teachers, and
they so desire, I devote much time to their training. They also
periodically attend seminars with other Yoga teachers as part
of their growth.

The ultimate test of a good teacher can only be measured in
how well you learn to do the exercises, provided, of course,
that you do your share of practicing. Unless you have a physical handicap, you will be able to perform most of the Yoga
positions. Most students in my classes do all the exercises
listed within six months. Except for those with special problems, all my students can execute the Intermediate Headstand
within three months—an accomplishment always accompanied by a great feeling of exultation.

You may not always find the teacher who is tuned in on
precisely your wave length, but you can learn from him just
the same. Do try to avoid the type so enamored of his own
body that he spends most of the class time posing in various
positions to show himself to his best advantage. While his
prowess may impress you, you won't learn much from him.

Empathy is an important quality in a Yoga instructor, too.
He should really understand the capacity and limitations of
his students. I once had a young instructor, possessed with
boundless energy, who worked his beginners' class of

middle-agers into a state of complete exhaustion. Beware of the teacher who urges you to try difficult advanced positions before you are ready for them, and be prepared to exercise your own common sense. In one beginners' class I attended, the instructor effortlessly assumed the Crow position and told us to try it. What most of the other students and I didn't know then was that the Crow is one of the very advanced positions which should be taught only to experienced students with highly developed coordination. Most of us went into the Crow and fell flat on our knees on the concrete floor. To sum up: Follow a teacher, but never blindly.

There are some teachers who give private lessons, but these are generally expensive. While they should be sought by the person suffering with a very specific physical problem, group lessons are preferable for the majority. A class should contain no more students than the teacher can supervise and work with individually. Group lessons are enjoyable, but if they are given in enormous groups it can become quite frustrating, especially when one has to strain to see what the teacher is demonstrating.

It is fun to share your interest in Yoga with others. I know one elderly lady who not only practices Yoga faithfully but has added new interest to her life and made new friends by attending Yoga lectures, meetings, and other activities that are available in New York City.

Today Yoga is taught in most large cities in the United States. Check the yellow pages for Yoga centers or with your local Y. There are also churches and synagogues that sponsor Yoga classes and schools that feature them as part of their adult education program. And you could go to a Yoga retreat or resort on your vacation.

If there is no Yoga class available where you live, take the initiative and organize one. Any of the above-mentioned institutions would probably be glad to sponsor a class if they were made aware of the interest in Yoga and its benefits. You could find a teacher through the nearest Yoga center or retreat.

There are many health clubs and resort hotels that because of popular request combine Yoga with their regular programs of calisthenics and machine exercises. But Yoga done haphazardly, either as part of other exercises or on an unscheduled basis, has little purpose or meaning.

My course is scientifically structured and designed to allow the student to experience readily evident benefits. After a six-week session, everyone reports a favorable change: improved flexibility and agility, awareness of body and mind, and an increase in endurance and energy. Sleeping better, feeling better, or looking better—something definite will have taken place to give the students incentive to continue. I teach beginners', intermediate, and advanced courses, so that Yoga can be firmly established as part of one's life.

Whether you're attending a class at the Y, the Unitarian Church Community House, or your neighbor's basement, be prepared to pay at least a nominal fee. There are some Yoga societies that maintain it is unspiritual to teach Yoga for money. They exist on contributions, and their teachers are not paid. However, human nature being what it is, people tend to value most that which they pay for, whether it be advice or Yoga lessons. People will not attend with the same regularity or put the same amount of effort into free lessons as they will into lessons that have been paid for—in advance. When lessons are paid for on a pay-as-you-go plan, it is too easy to become lazy or discouraged and give up before you have begun to experience the benefits of Yoga. The majority of my students who stick with their first course continue in the ensuing courses. The sad thing is that the ones who do drop out of the first course are the very ones who would benefit the most. The overweight, overnervous, most uncoordinated and inflexible give the excuse, "Yoga may be for some, but not for me." It is, however, for everyone who gives it and himself a chance.

Having read this far, you understand that it isn't necessary to deprive yourself of your everyday pleasures in order to practice Yoga. Yoga demands no martyrs. But although you won't be required to give up what you now consider your fun, as you seriously practice Yoga your ideas of fun may change. Everywhere people are engaged in a feverish pursuit of happiness, constantly seeking excitement and stimulation in purposeless activity, drugs, alcohol, and sex. "The world is a hopeless mess, and we're all doomed. Accept the futility and rottenness of life, and get your kicks where you can," they say. After a while all the thrills begin to pall, but the dissatisfaction remains. External stimulation may provide momentary diversion, but the genuine source of all pleasure comes from within. That is why Yoga is so valuable—it can help you to discover yourself. It can lead you to the sources of inner strength and serenity. Satisfaction with yourself can enable you to derive real pleasure from whatever you do—your work, your play, your relationships with other people. The experience of Yoga is a pleasure in itself, but it will also open new doors to pleasures in other phases of your life.

You will probably find that your intellectual powers have improved, and you will derive new enjoyment from stimulating your mind. Your capacity to absorb complex subjects like philosophy and science may increase.

You may eliminate certain habits and tastes that are incompatible with Yoga, like smoking and drinking hard liquor. Others you may modify. I used to be an inveterate bridge player, but now I find the tension that accompanies most bridge games and the relaxation of Yoga just don't mix. I still play an occasional game of bridge, but only with a partner who, like me, plays for pleasure, not blood.

Through Yoga you can experience a subtle change in your character—more patience, understanding, and honesty toward others and yourself. Yoga can help foster self-confidence and a more mature attitude. Those who feel secure about their own worth as human beings do not have to frantically race to keep up with the Joneses financially or socially.

In the subtle way that Yoga works to change your outlook on life, it can help you to better appreciate your family, the friends who are true friends, and, most importantly, your own company. Many people are alone, but no one needs to be lonely. Solitude is not loneliness. Loneliness is a state of dissatisfaction which one may feel even in the midst of people. Yoga can become a friend and a companion to the alone and to the lonely. None experience greater solitude than the blind. Sally is completely blind and lives alone except for her Seeing Eye dog, Tommy. They both come to class. While Sally does the exercises, Tommy observes the class and, during relaxation, falls asleep. Eyes are not necessary for meditation, and Sally was able to grasp the vision within by concentrating on the third eye. She learned to "see," not externally but internally. Yoga can help everyone to see the internal vision, so necessary in times of loneliness and despair.

Certainly no one can ignore the troubled times we live in. Every morning's newspapers bring fresh accounts of wars, riots, and social miseries. Our own sense of frustration is deepened because we personally are able to do little or nothing about these events. Yoga can provide a refuge to help us maintain our own internal equilibrium and levelheadedness in the midst of external turbulence. We turn inward to build our own strength and peace.

This does not mean that you use Yoga to cut yourself off

from the world. Rather, Yoga helps you fortify yourself so you can function efficiently and calmly in the midst of general and personal upheaval.

Just as nature has fashioned the individual with the potential for good health, so has she fashioned him with the potential for joy. Unhappiness and tragedy come uninvited, but happiness must be sought. Often a person must train himself to recognize joy when it is present, or else he will only realize it was there once it is gone. Through Yoga you can learn how to feel happy *now;* how not to dwell on the past or fill your time with worries and daydreams of the future, but to truly live only in the present.

You can find enjoyment in every day of life with Yoga. It has been around for thousands of years, giving new life to those who take advantage of what it has to offer. I honestly believe it is the wave of the future. In spite of reversals, the world is moving forward. Eventually, more and more people will come to choose Yoga as the most reasonable path to follow. Now discover Yoga yourself. It makes common sense.

EXERCISES

BASIC PROGRAM

Yoga and Practice

HERE IS a basic program for beginners and intermediates. Many people who begin Yoga and thoroughly enjoy it do not continue because they do not understand how to practice.* They set the wrong goals for practice and then give up when they cannot reach them. The only goal in Yoga is awareness.

*To facilitate home practice we have made a cassette tape for use in conjunction with this book. To obtain a copy, please send $6.95 in check or money order to Yoga for Long Island, 965 Willis Avenue, Albertson, New York 11507. The price includes tax and mailing costs.

Yoga is a process of becoming aware of your body, its functions, and its life force.

Practice should be consistent: you strive to practice every day, but you understand that there are days when circumstances prevent practice, and so you do not allow guilt to come from these unavoidably missed days.

You try to allow one hour to practice this basic program. But when you do not have an hour, remember it is better to do a few postures slowly, thoroughly, and with utmost concentration, than to try for every posture. On days when you have more time you can enjoy doing the whole program or even some special postures. On days with little time select a few postures and work for perfection.

Practice Plan #1: 30-40 minutes

Spinal Roll
At least one standing pose, such as the Triangle
At least one sitting pose, such as the Alternate Leg Stretch
Shoulderstand
Fish
Cobra or Locust or Bow
Breathing Exercises
Total Relaxation

Practice Plan #2: 20-30 minutes

Spinal Roll
One or more postures from the Basic Program on which you are working specially hard or
One or more postures you want to learn from the Special Exercise Section
Total Relaxation

Practice Plan #3: 20 minutes and up

Spinal Roll
Whichever postures your common sense and developing body awareness tell you to do
Total Relaxation

Practice Time and Space

It is good to have a regular practice time. The morning is best, as you will start your day off vibrant with all your body, mind, and emotions really working. Furthermore, the stomach is really empty, which makes practice much better. However, practice is more difficult in the morning, in that the body contracts during sleep. If you prefer that time to exercise, a warm shower or bath to loosen up will help.

Some people prefer evening practice, to relax them after their day. This, too, is fine. You should not eat for at least two hours before exercising, so you will have to plan your evening meal accordingly. If you eat after practice, wait one half-hour.

Of course, some days you might fit Yoga into another available time slot. But whichever time you choose should be a quiet time of your own, and you should make your practice space truly inviting to you.

When you're just beginning, make sure all furniture is out of the way. A miscarried Shoulderstand has been known to result in a broken lamp or bruised shin. Once you become adept at Yoga you'll need only a very small practice area and won't have to concern yourself with the fragility of your surroundings.

Dress

Keep body distractions out—no hair that has to be adjusted or pushed from the eyes, no jewelry to get in the way, etc.

If you choose to practice clothed, leotards are very flattering and professional-looking. I urge you, however, to wear as little as possible, as this allows you to be much more in touch with your body.

Use of Your Senses

Yoga is a process of harmony. Your mind, your body, your emotions, and your spirit function in healthy harmony. You must use all your senses in practice. Keep your eyes open and keep watching the body movement. Use mirrors if you can. Use your hands to feel body movement, even though in the completed posture your hands will be aligned according to the instructions. Feel with every other part of your body as well. Listen to your breathing: it will become an indicator of many things concerning proper practice. Keep checking that you have your body properly aligned as you move into each pose and as you change poses.

Breathing Practice

You may practice your breathing at a different time from your practice of postures—for reasons of either time or relaxation. You may practice breathing immediately before postures. This has the added advantage of making your body fully oxygenated and relaxed as you go into the postures. If you choose to practice breathing after the postures but before Total Relaxation, you should rest between the postures and the breathing. Your heart and pulse rate should return to normal before you proceed from postures to breathing work.

All breathing that accompanies postures is done through the nose. Exhale through the mouth only when specified. Never hold an inhale or an exhale longer than you are ready to—it is better to take an extra breath.

General Hints

Do not be upset if you do not understand all the details of the directions for the postures. As you practice with growing awareness you will understand more and more. The pictures are of completed postures. You are to go only as far as you can and use the pictures for direction. Concentrate on working both sides evenly and on moving slowly and gracefully.

Most likely, you are beginning Yoga with a body that is out of condition. Therefore, regard your body as unused territory that will need patient cultivation. You will be setting to work joints, muscles, tendons, and ligaments that have long lain dormant. Be gentle, and don't expect the impossible right away. You will have to condition your body slowly by stretching muscles and loosening joints that until now have had little or no exercise at all.

Eventually you will reach your goal of firmness and flexibility, but straining and jerking your body won't get you there. Don't worry about reaching the ultimate position at the beginning. Your body will benefit from even the partial execution of a hold or exercise. Even when you think you're not getting anywhere, your body is proving the opposite by stretching a little at a time. Provide your body with the incentive, and it will do the rest.

While you shouldn't strain, you should work to the utmost of your capacity. When you have reached a plateau in a position, go on to a more advanced stage of the exercise. For example, in the Alternate Leg Stretch, when you can grasp your calf, start trying to do the exercise holding on to your ankle. Yoga should present a constant challenge to the body.

You will experience aches and discomforts in various parts of your body until it becomes accustomed to being stretched, even when you attempt new positions after doing Yoga for some time. This is natural and will soon pass away.

When you practice your exercises, focus all your attention on Yoga. Don't think about how you're going to pay the insurance premium, why your stock keeps going down, or what to serve at your dinner party on Saturday night. Think only about Yoga, and let all your thoughts be graceful ones. Yoga demands the cooperation of a good imagination. You may not be moving with all the grace and poise of a sleek, shiny cat, but imagine that you are. Pretty soon you will be.

This will probably be one of the few times during your fast-paced day that you will not be rushing. And at first, slowing down won't come easily. Be conscious that each exercise should be done slowly. Go into it slowly, and remember to come out of it just as slowly.

Be aware that you are working only for yourself in what may be the most beneficial undertaking of your life.

STANDING EXERCISES

Spinal Roll (to warm up)

Sit cross-legged. Reach for your feet or ankles and pull them close to your thighs. Bring your head forward and let yourself roll back by swinging your feet overhead. And then roll forward with the momentum. Again roll all the way back, touching your knees to the floor if you can, and roll forward. Continue. If you find this too difficult as yet, try a modified Spinal Roll, pressing both knees to the chest and clasping your arms around the knees. Repeat this about ten times. Keep your spine curled and think of yourself as a rubber ball bouncing back and forth. You will loosen every vertebra in your spinal column. When you have finished, lie down and relax for a few minutes until your breathing is normalized.

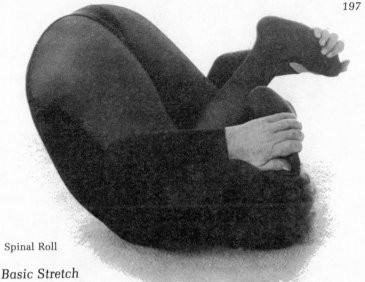

Spinal Roll

Basic Stretch

Stand with your feet in a V position with the heels together for proper balance. During the count of eight, simultaneously inhale, slowly lift your arms out sideways, palms outward, then over your head, and rise up onto your toes. Exhale. Clasp one of your thumbs, keeping your elbows straight and your head between your arms, and stretch. Hold the stretch, breathing normally for an eight count. Inhale deeply. While exhaling, lower your arms, palms down, and lower your heels to the floor to the count of eight.

Gradually increase inhalation and exhalation to a ten count and the holding period by five counts at a time until you can hold for a twenty count.

Perform three times.

BENEFITS

This overall stretch relaxes you by breaking through internal and external tensions.

It promotes both a general feeling of youthfulness and a youthful appearance.

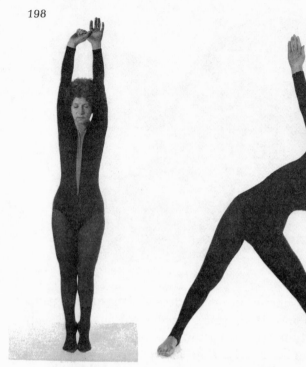

Basic Stretch   Triangle Pose

It increases your sense of balance and poise.
It stretches your spine.
It helps increase coordination.
It acts to totally invigorate you.

Triangle Pose

Place the feet three to three and a half feet apart and parallel
to each other. The arms should be at shoulder level with the
palms down.

Simultaneously move the left hip directly to the left and
slide the right hand as far down the right leg as you can
without bringing the torso or pelvic area forward. Gaze up at
the left hand.

Hold the position, breathing normally in and out ten times. Exhale as you return to start.

Repeat on the other side.

It increases balance.

It tones and strengthens legs, waist, abdomen, hips, chest, shoulders, and arms.

It increases lateral flexibility of the spine.

Dancer's Pose

Stand straight with your arms at your sides. Move your right foot forward slightly, placing all your weight on it. Slowly bend your left leg behind you and press it firmly against your body with your left hand, keeping your thighs together. At this point, straighten your body and establish your balance. Inhale, raise your right arm straight up over your head, stretch your body upward, bring your head back, and pull your left foot up toward your back. Exhale. Breathing normally, hold the stretch for a ten count. Inhale. Exhaling, simultaneously lower your arm and foot.

Perform this exercise balancing two times on the right foot and two times on the left.

A good way to practice for this position is to lift one leg and bounce on the other, keeping the sole of your foot flat on the floor.

Throughout the exercise, concentrate on the foot that bears your weight.

If you find it too difficult to perform this exercise, until your balance has improved, you may lightly rest the side supporting your weight against a wall.

Once you have mastered the above, continue to the more advanced movements of this position. Do not lower your arm and foot in the first position. Tilt your body forward and clasp both hands around your ankle and extend your leg as far as possible.

Think of it as a ballet movement. Breathe normally and move forward until your torso is in line with the floor. Hold for a ten count.

Slowly straighten your body. Unclasp and lower your leg. Repeat on the other side.

BENEFITS

The Dancer's Pose is an intense stretch for the spine, back, and shoulders, relieving backaches and tension in the back and shoulders.

It works to improve the entire figure.

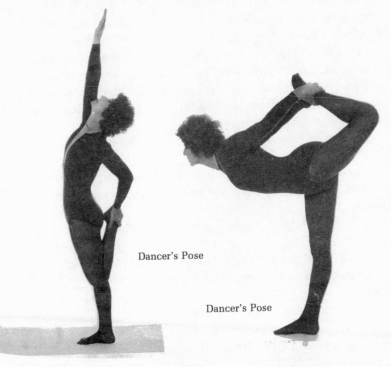

Dancer's Pose

Dancer's Pose

It develops the chest and beautifies the bustline.

It improves posture.

It aids in attaining poise, grace, and coordination for the whole body.

Standing Twist

Stand straight, with your feet about twelve inches apart. Turn wrists until fingertips point upwards. Extend your arms straight out sideways at shoulder level. Inhale. Exhaling, twist your body slowly to the left, keeping your feet flat on the floor, until you are facing the back wall, if possible. Breathing normally, hold for a ten count. Inhaling, slowly twist back. Without lowering the arms, repeat two more times. Lower the arms. Do three times to the right.

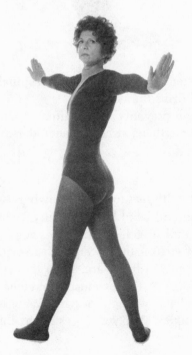

Standing Twist

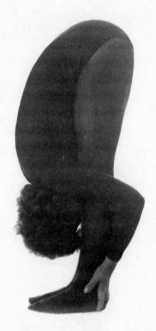

Head Knee Bend

BENEFITS

This is an excellent exercise for achieving spinal flexibility.
It reduces and firms the waistline.
It eliminates and prevents a spare tire.
It firms and strengthens arms and shoulders.

Head Knee Bend

Stand straight, with feet together. Slowly raise your arms
straight overhead and bend back carefully, tightening your
buttocks. Inhale and stretch up. Exhale as you bend forward
from the waist, stretching the lower back and bringing the rib
cage toward the thighs in an arc. Keep the weight evenly
distributed on both feet, the leg muscles stretched and lifted.
Firmly grasp the back of whatever part of your legs you can
reach, calves or ankles. Keep your legs straight. Inhale. Exhale

and come further into the position by bending the elbows and bringing your chest toward your knees. Try not to round the lower back. Breathing normally, hold for a ten count.

Release the hold on the legs and let your body dangle loosely like a rag doll. Straighten up, piling one vertebra onto the next very slowly, pushing the small of the back to the ceiling and contracting the abdomen. The head, neck, and arms are limp.

Repeat twice.

BENEFITS

This is an overall firmer and beautifier for the entire body.

It firms and slenderizes the hips.

It stretches and strengthens the ligaments in the back, neck, and legs.

The completed movement assures superb flexibility of the entire spine.

SITTING EXERCISES

Gracefully cross the legs and come to a sitting position, placing the hands by the thighs for support. Since much of our Yoga work is done in one of the cross-legged poses, please read the entire section so that you understand the Half Lotus and the Lotus Pose and how to practice to attain them.

Half Lotus/Full Lotus Pose

Extend your legs in front of you. Hold on to your right foot with both hands and place the sole against the inside of your left thigh. Bend your left knee and gently lift up your leg to rest it on your right thigh. Make an effort to bring both knees to the floor and to sit as straight as possible. Alternate sides.

You should only attempt the Full Lotus when you are

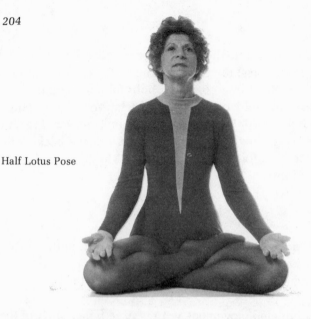

Half Lotus Pose

totally comfortable and can bring your knees to the floor in the Half Lotus described above.

To do the Full Lotus, bending your knee, hold on to your foot with both hands, and lift it gently but firmly to lie as high as possible on the opposite thigh. Repeat with the other leg, so that each foot rests on the thigh of the opposite leg.

In the beginning, hold the posture for only a few seconds, gradually increasing the time to one minute or longer, and eventually achieving a comfortable position to be assumed during meditation.

You will find one leg to be much more pliable and coopera-tive than the other, but to arrive at perfect physical balance of the body, you must work equally, or perhaps more, with the other leg.

If your knees are very tight, and neither position is possible as yet, practice the Leg Bounce whenever possible. Extend your legs in front of you. Gently pick up your right foot and guide it over to rest on top of your left thigh, as high into the

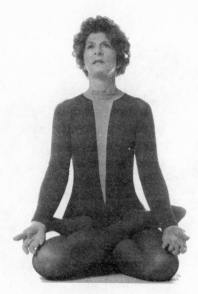

Full Lotus Pose

groin as possible. Don't be dismayed if your right knee is way up in the air. Hold your foot with your left hand. Placing your right hand on top of your right knee, bounce it gently. Reverse sides. Don't force or strain. As your legs become more flexible, try the Half Lotus, then the Full Lotus. The Lotus can take many, many months to achieve, but remember—it's the process, not the end result, that counts.

BENEFITS

It makes the legs more shapely. I've found that the Lotus Pose beautifies the legs more than any other posture. Heavy legs become slimmer, and skinny legs fill out.

It firms the thighs.

It strengthens the ankles.

It restores elasticity to legs, hips, and ankles.

By improving the blood circulation, it helps prevent arthritis and rheumatism, and greatly relieves any existing joint disease.

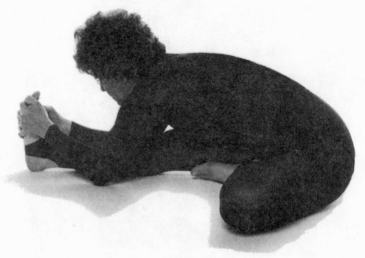

Alternate Leg Stretch

Alternate Leg Stretch

This exercise is the guideline for determining the flexibility of the spine, which is the prerequisite for all the following exercises. Once the spine is flexible, everything else will fall into line. You don't have to strain, pull, jerk, or fidget, for while you are just holding the position, the spine will stretch itself, with the effects extending the whole spinal column. Although there may be some initial discomfort, it will soon disappear. Sit straight with legs in front of you. With both hands, pick up your left foot and place the heel in the perineum with the sole against the right thigh. Always handle your limbs gently to avoid discomfort. Keep both knees on the floor, if possible, and the back straight. Place your hands in front of you, palms down, and clasp one thumb. Take a deep breath, simultaneously lifting your arms, with the elbows straight, above your head. Lean back slightly, and stretch

from the waist. Exhaling, come forward over your right leg.
Firmly clasp, with thumbs on top, whatever part of your leg
you can reach—knee, calf or ankle. Bending elbows outward
and keeping shoulders back and down, gently slide your torso
forward, bringing the rib cage toward the thigh. Do not permit
the lower back to become rounded, even if you can move
forward only a couple of inches at the beginning. Breathing
normally, continue to stretch, sinking into the position; but
do not strain. Hold for ten seconds, gradually increasing to
twenty seconds. Inhaling, sit up slowly, gracefully sliding
your hands up your legs, and without stopping, move into the
reverse repetition of this posture.

Perform three times on each side. To do the advanced
position, place your foot on top of the thigh as in the Half
Lotus; the knee must touch the floor.

BENEFITS

The Alternate Leg Stretch is one of the best positions for
restoring flexibility, elasticity, and youthfulness to any spine
in any condition.

The hold benefits the legs as much as the back, by stretching the muscles, ligaments, and tendons.

It relieves stiffness and tension, especially in the back of the
legs. It firms the entire body, especially legs, thighs, buttocks,
hips, and abdomen.

Inner Thigh Stretch

Sit erect. Place the soles of your feet together. Interlock your
fingers and place your hands under your feet. Pull your feet
toward you. Do not allow the spine to round—keep pushing
the chest through the arms to keep it straight. Inhale deeply.
Exhaling gently with steady pressure, push your knees
toward the floor. Don't be afraid to push down as far as

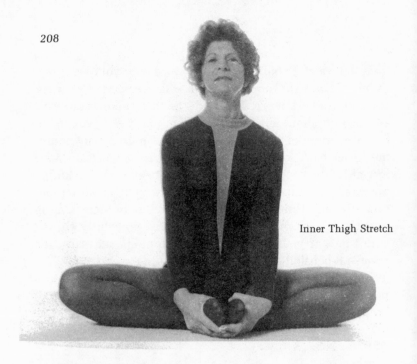

Inner Thigh Stretch

possible. Breathing normally, hold the extreme position for ten seconds and release.

Perform three times.

BENEFITS

Prepares knees and ankle joints for Lotus Pose.
Tones and tightens inner thighs.
Straightens spine.

Straighten legs, place hands on thighs, press the chin into the jugular notch. Contract the abdomen and very slowly lie down. As you press the legs firmly against the floor, you will strengthen the lower back and tighten all visceral organs.

Hollow Breath

As you lie down on your back, close your eyes. Pull up your legs and rest the soles of your feet flat on the floor. Rest your

fingertips lightly on your abdomen. Inhale as slowly as possible, pushing the abdomen up and out sideways as far as it will
go. Exhale as slowly as possible, contracting the abdomen at
the same speed. When the breath is completely exhaled,
firmly contract the abdominal muscles, push the small of the
back flat against the floor, contract the buttocks so that the
pelvis is tilted up slightly and the abdominal cavity is hol-
lowed. Hold out your breath for eight seconds. Relax the
abdomen completely before inhaling again.

Perform eight times. Gradually increase the time you hold
out your breath to ten, fifteen, and, as you gain proficiency,
twenty seconds.

BENEFITS

This technique induces calmness. Practice it any time you
are suffering from stress or agitation.

This is one of the techniques used in natural childbirth to
promote complete relaxation of the abdominal area and of the
entire nervous system.

It acts as a refresher to relieve fatigue.

It rids the body of toxins and wastes.

It firms the abdominal muscles and is especially good for
strengthening the abdominal wall after childbirth or surgery.

It strengthens the inner organs and the muscles of the lower
back.

Shoulderstand

Legs are straight together, arms close to the body, palms of
the hands down. Pressing arms and hands against the floor,
raise your legs, while contracting the abdomen. When your
legs are perpendicular to the floor, inhale quickly, raising the
hips and buttocks off the floor and placing your hands on the
lower spine for support. Exhale. If this is too difficult as yet,
roll your knees to your forehead, as in the Spinal Roll, placing

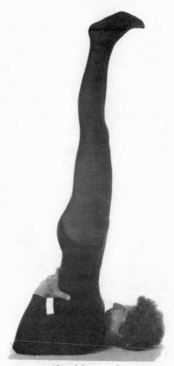

Shoulderstand

your hands on the buttocks and lower back for support, and then straighten the legs.

Whichever way you get up, gradually move your hands up your spine toward the floor and move your elbows closer together, eventually reaching the extreme position, with legs and body straight as a candle. Thighs, inner knees, ankles, and soles should touch, with legs and spine stretching toward the ceiling. Press your chin into your jugular notch. The feet are flexed and relaxed. Work up to holding the position for three minutes, breathing normally.

As your spine becomes stronger, try moving your hands toward the floor and interlocking them as pictured in the Plough. In the ultimate position, the body rests entirely on the shoulders, with the chin pressed into the collarbone and the back of the neck soft against the floor.

Keep in mind that holding the body in any degree of inversion is beneficial. If you can't straighten your body at first, hold it at any angle at which you can support yourself with your hands. As your spine becomes stronger, it will straighten further.

If you cannot lift your hips off the floor, practice lying in a doorway over the threshold. By holding on to the side of the doorway, you will be able to lift your hips off the floor.

Two excellent exercises for firming the legs that can be done in the inverted position of the Shoulderstand are the Slow Bicycle and the Scissors. Slow Bicycle—Slowly rotate your legs as if you were pushing the pedals of a bike. Scissors—Slowly open your legs wide to the sides and bring them together in the action of the blades of a pair of scissors opening and closing.

If you are having difficulty with the Shoulderstand, practice the Back Push-Up from the Special Postures Section.

BENEFITS

The blood is able to flow freely through the entire body, stimulating organs and glands. Improved circulation helps relieve pain of varicose veins. The heart is relieved of the difficulty of pumping to the upper body against the force of gravity.

Increased blood supply to the head improves the complexion.

The spine is strengthened.

The stepped-up flow of blood to the brain combats fatigue and tones up the nervous system.

The visceral organs are relieved of the constant pull of gravity. This often helps correct digestive disorders.

Pressing the chin into the jugular notch can stimulate and

massage the thyroid gland as an aid to normalizing weight and promoting overall health.

Rollout

To come out of the Shoulderstand, fold your legs close to your body and open your hands flat on the floor. As a beginner, you may bend your knees. Inhale. Exhaling, slowly lower your legs all the way to the floor. To prevent your head from rising off the floor while rolling out, arch your neck and upper back, especially in the beginning. As you become more advanced, keep the shoulders relaxed and the back of the neck soft on the floor, and tighten the abdominal and leg muscles as well as the buttocks. As you achieve control of your body, try to keep the legs straight and the small of the back on the floor from the second the entire spine has rolled onto the floor until you have finished lowering your legs. While rolling out, pause for a few seconds with the weight on each vertebra. As soon as your legs touch the floor, let your feet flop open and your body soften and relax onto the floor, and breathe deeply.

BENEFITS

This gradual lowering movement exercises, stimulates, and massages the entire spine, working out each vertebra and effecting perfect spinal health.

Rollout

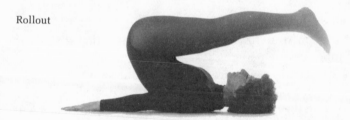

Plough

You may go into the Plough from the Shoulderstand by keeping the spine straight and lowering the legs toward the floor behind the head. Or, if you have rolled out of the Shoulderstand, you may lie with the legs straight together, arms next to your body, and the palms of your hands down. Pressing your arms and palms against the floor, raise your legs, keeping them straight. As in the Shoulderstand, concentrate on tightening your leg and abdominal muscles. Inhale. Exhale and continue straightening the spine, pushing the bones of the buttocks up toward the ceiling and bringing the toes toward the floor. Breathing normally, increase holding time to two minutes. You may interlock your hands.

To straighten the spine, walk your feet toward your head, pushing the shoulders into the floor and the coccyx toward the ceiling.

To roll out, bend your knees close to your head and place palms and arms flat against the floor. Straightening the legs as you come down, lower the body as from the Shoulderstand.

When you are beginning the Plough and your feet don't reach the floor as yet, support your back and fold your knees toward your head. Straighten your legs little by little as your spine gains flexibility.

Plough

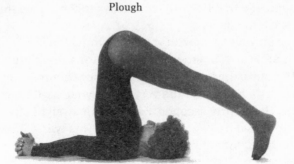

Fish Pose

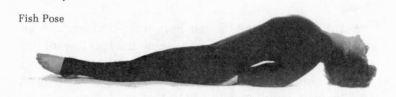

BENEFITS

A healthful conditioning pressure is applied to the abdominal and pelvic organs.

The spine is stretched for maximum flexibility and rejuvenation.

Dorsal muscles are strengthened.

Blood circulation is improved, resulting in a lovelier complexion.

The Plough firms the hips, thighs, and abdomen, while helping to subtract inches from those areas.

It can often provide almost immediate relief from tension and headache.

Arthritis and backache sufferers have reported the greatest relief with this posture.

Fish Pose

This pose should be performed after rolling out of the Plough. It will relieve all tension by stretching the spine from concave to convex.

Lie on your back, with your legs straight in front of you and your arms at your sides. Place your arms straight under you, with your palms on the floor. Lift your shoulders and upper back in an arch, with the very top of your head touching the floor. Hold thirty seconds. Feel how the weight of your body is supported by your lower arms. Do this twice. Then do it a third time, inhaling as you arch up. Hold ten seconds, and exhale.

Extreme Fish Pose

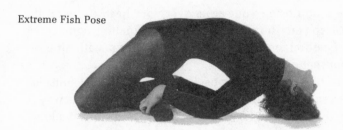

BENEFITS

This posture is of great cosmetic value to both men and women, preventing crepy neck and double chins by firming the muscles. It can also improve any existing unattractive condition.

The thyroid gland is stimulated.

This exercise acts as an overall tonic to the nervous system.

Extreme Fish Pose

Lie on your back, cross your legs and fold them under you. Hold on to your feet or, if possible, your ankles. Arch the upper part of your body as in the Single Fish Pose, simultaneously pulling your feet under your buttocks. Now arch your thighs and hips, and bring your knees to touch the floor. This position really sounds and looks more complicated than it is. It can be achieved by most intermediate students.

Practice as in the Fish Pose.

BENEFITS

In addition to the benefits of the Fish Pose:

It firms the thighs and hips.

It strengthens and rejuvenates the feet.

It relieves tension throughout the spine.

If your back and abdominal musculature is fairly strong, to move into a sitting position for the next exercise, straighten your legs and bring your arms over your head to lie on the floor. Clasp your thumb, inhale deeply. Exhaling, come into a sitting position, head between the upper arms, without moving your feet off the floor.

If you have weak lower-back and/or abdominal muscles, exercise caution until they are strengthened. Use this way of sitting up: Bend one leg, clasp both hands around the knee, and sit up, exhaling.

Complete Leg Stretch

The Complete Leg Stretch is a variation on the Alternate Leg Stretch, which you performed earlier in your practice session to loosen up your tight muscles. As you do this now, you will see how your body has gained in flexibility from the preceding movements.

Sit erect, with legs extended straight in front of you and hands on your thighs. Slowly raise both arms straight in front of you until they are above your head. Clasp your thumb, stretch, and inhale. Exhaling, dive slowly, stretching the lower back and leading with the rib cage. Grip firmly whatever part of your legs you can reach: calves, ankles, or feet. Bending your elbows, pull your torso forward. Hold your

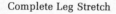

Complete Leg Stretch

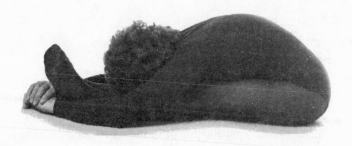

extreme position, breathing normally, for twenty seconds.
Do three times.

BENEFITS

The Complete Leg Stretch provides an intense stretch to the
spinal column and legs, strengthening and restoring elasticity to all the muscles involved.

It loosens the hamstrings and the muscles in back of knees
and thighs.

It is a powerful aid in firming the legs.

It helps reduce the waist, abdomen, and hips.

A word before going on. Coming up are the three classic
Yoga positions performed on the abdomen, and they are the
most strenuous exercises—the Cobra, the Locust, and the
Bow. I must admit they're not so much fun as the others, but
they certainly should not be neglected. For although they
require the utmost diligence, these are three of the most important Yoga exercises, because they work directly on both
the inner organs and the outer body to restore and maintain
complete physical health. Be sure to allow two minutes between these exercises to relax and to repeat deep breathing.

A graceful way to move from your sitting position to a
prone position is to bend your legs and bring them both to one
side. Place your hands firmly on the floor in front of you, and
swing yourself around to lie on your abdomen.

Cobra

Breathe normally.

Lie on your stomach. Place your arms directly under your
chest, with fingertips facing straight ahead. If this is too
difficult for you, move your hands up to twelve inches for-

ward, so that you will be able to rise into the position as follows: In a succession of flowing movements, lift up your chin, roll back your head, stretch your torso forward, and raise your shoulders. Keeping your pelvis on the floor and your head back, continue pushing yourself up as slowly as possible, until your arms are straight. Hold your extreme position twenty seconds, concentrating on shifting all your weight onto your arms without allowing your shoulders to hunch or become tense. At the same time, tighten your buttocks and roll your abdomen into the floor. Keep gazing farther and farther back on the ceiling. The feet, knees and thighs should be touching, but if you have a weak lower back, let the legs separate slightly. Keep your navel firmly pressed into the floor and don't raise higher. Hold ten seconds at first, gradually increasing to thirty.

Bend your elbows and slowly lower your body, keeping your head back as long as possible. Your chin should be the last part of your body to reach the floor. Turn your head to the side and relax. Perform twice.

If you find the straight-arm position uncomfortable, you can start by placing your hands parallel to each other under your chest. Use your hands to push yourself up slowly, keeping the elbows bent and against the body for support. Hold the position to your capacity. Come down the same way, with your arms supporting you.

BENEFITS

The Cobra stretches all the vertebrae, especially those of the upper back and neck, promoting flexibility and generally toning the spine and sympathetic nervous system.

Accumulated tension in the upper back and neck is relieved. Posture is improved.

All the inner organs, including the sex glands, are massaged, stimulating the action of these organs for general good health and sexual vitality.

Muscles in the abdomen, bust, and chest are firmed.

Symptoms of arthritis are relieved.

The Cobra provides fresh vitality. Yet it induces sleep in cases of insomnia.

Locust Pose

Lie on your stomach, with your arms at your sides, chin on the floor and feet together. Make fists and bring your entire arms under you with your fists under your thighs, so that your body is supported by your arms. Your fists can be up or down, whichever way provides the best balance. Inhale. Keeping your chin on the floor and both feet together, quickly raise both legs off the floor as high and straight as you can. Exhale and hold eight seconds, breathing normally. Exhale and lower to the count of five.

Do it twice, gradually increasing the hold to twenty seconds. Relax completely and breathe deeply.

In the beginning try to lift your legs only five inches off the floor. Hold for an eight count and lower slowly.

Cobra

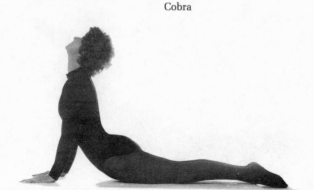

The muscles of the lower body and the arms are subjected to strong tension, resulting in firming of the upper arms, abdomen, hips, buttocks, and thighs.

The sex organs and glands are stimulated.

The Locust works on the lower-back area, with emphasis on the sacroiliac. The visceral organs and glands are stimulated, helping to relieve digestive disorders.

Bow Pose

If you have lower-back problems, do not attempt this position until you strengthen your back.

Lie on your stomach, thighs apart and chin on the floor. Bring your heels up toward your back. Reach back and firmly grip your ankles. Raise your head, shoulders, and chest off the floor. Then lift your legs as high as possible, arching into a perfect bow. Hold ten seconds. Lower your knees, then the upper part of your body, and finally let go of your legs. Turn your head to the side. Relax and breathe deeply.

Locust Pose

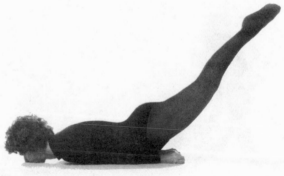

Do three times, gradually increasing the hold to twenty seconds.

For variation, rock back and forth slowly. If you are advanced, try to bring your thighs together. If you can't raise both legs, lift one leg at a time. This will strengthen your leg and back muscles, so that eventually you will be able to perform the Bow with both legs.

BENEFITS

The Bow strengthens and develops the entire spine, resulting in complete elasticity.

It firms the entire body, with emphasis on the upper arms, bust, hips, buttocks, and thighs.

It improves posture.

It helps relieve menstrual disorders and lower-back pain.

Many of my students report that this exercise gives complete relief from physical and mental tension.

Bow Pose

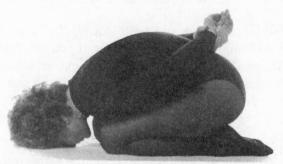

Embryo Pose

Embryo Pose

This is a counterpose for the Cobra, Locust, and Bow.

Place your hands palms down next to your shoulders. Lift your head and push up and back slowly on your straight arms. As you push up, intensely stretch your trunk and spine, until you are sitting on your heels. Imagine you are a cat stretching every part of its body. Let your head drop in front of your knees. Rest your hands palms up by your hips. Relax in this pose for one minute. Rise slowly.

BENEFITS

This is an excellent stimulation for the feet.
It can be used any time for relaxation.
It relieves tension in the lower back.

The Yoga Headstand is often referred to as "King of Asanas" because of all its beneficial results and for the overwhelming sense of satisfaction you will experience upon achieving it. Some find it easy; others, quite difficult. But the Yoga Headstand is not an acrobatic feat. It can be mastered by anyone. The greatest obstacle to achieving it is the fear of falling, which can be conquered with patience and practice. Following are the three positions of the Headstand.

Dolphin

1. Kneel and sit on your heels. Lean forward and place your forearms on the floor. Interlock your fingers and place your hands on the floor with palms toward you.

2. Fit the back of your head into the palms of your hands, with the top of your forehead resting on the floor. Keep your elbows as close together as possible. The two elbows and the clasped hands/head should form the three points of a triangle which acts as the foundation for the inverted positions.

3. Concentrate on distributing your weight on your forearms. Push up on your toes, lifting your body and straightening your legs. At this point your body has formed an arch.

4. Walk in toward yourself, bringing your knees as close to your chest as you can.

5. Hold twenty seconds. Raise your head slowly and return to kneeling position.

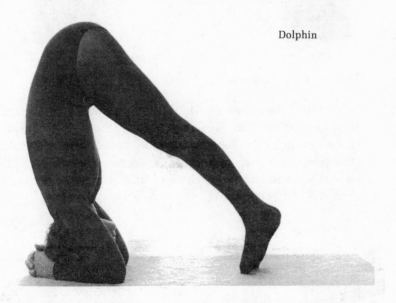

Dolphin

Intermediate Headstand

Headstand

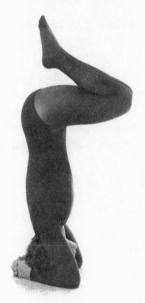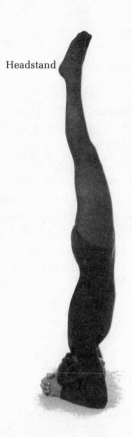

Intermediate Headstand

6. What you must now do is shift your weight from your feet to your forearms so that you walk into the Headstand. Raise one leg, then the other, keeping both legs folded. Hold this position ten seconds, gradually increasing your time. Do not attempt to straighten the legs until you are completely balanced and confident.

Headstand

7. Slowly straighten your knees and raise your legs in a straight line.

8. To come out of the Headstand, slowly fold your legs to the Intermediate Position. Roll down to rest on your knees. Do not pick up your head for at least thirty seconds, so that the blood can flow back normally. Then lie on your back and relax.

Hold the Headstand for three minutes, increasing to ten minutes. Remember, do not be in a hurry to achieve the full Headstand.

I advise caution in learning to perform this pose, because this is one Yoga position in which you can hurt yourself if you are not careful. Do not advance until you are completely confident that you have mastered the preliminary steps. Although there is little chance of hurting yourself in the rolled-up position, when you practice without assistance, make sure you're on a soft surface, or else surround yourself with pillows. Don't attempt the Headstand against a wall, because you can injure yourself, you can't attain the curled-up position, and you will have a false sense of security.

BENEFITS

I believe the psychological benefits of the Headstand are as important as the physical, because the ability to achieve and hold the position gives you a tremendous feeling of accomplishment and pride.

The complete inversion of the body increases the flow of blood to the brain, revitalizing you and stimulating your mental faculties.

It stimulates the thyroid, pineal, and pituitary glands.

It acts as a tonic for the entire nervous system.

Yogis consider the increased circulation to the scalp to be a preventive of gray hair, baldness, and wrinkles.

The complexion is improved.

It helps relieve symptoms of varicose veins.

It is said to retard the aging process by reversing the effects of gravity.

Complete Relaxation

I recommend that you always end your practice session with the Complete Relaxation. You can also do it any time you feel tense or fatigued.

Lie on your back, with your arms resting next to you, palms of your hands up, and legs straight and loose (the feet may turn out). Close your eyes, and completely let go of your body. Until you are accustomed to the art of Complete Relaxation, you will have to order your body to relax, command it to go limp, and visualize all the tension flowing out of your body. Let your breath come and go naturally. Try to detach yourself from your body and mind.

Now direct all your concentration on your feet—the toes, soles, heels, ankles, and insteps—shutting out all other thoughts. Relax the feet, all the muscles, tendons, and ligaments within.

Work upward now, going through the same process of relaxing the entire lower body—feet, calves, thighs, hips, waist, and lower back.

Relax the inner organs as well as the anal sphincter, buttocks, and abdominal muscles.

Now forget about the lower part of your body and concentrate on the area from the waist to the shoulders. Mentally travel upward and relax every vertebra of your spine. Relax the torso and shoulders.

Next, concentrate only on the hands and arms, slowly relaxing and letting the hands and arms lie loose, as if detached from the body.

Relax the neck, throat, and head next. Feel your face become soft, relaxed, and beautiful. Relax the chin, mouth, cheeks, and ears. Relax the nose, eyeballs, and eyelids. Relax the forehead, temples, and scalp.

Imagine that your whole body is very heavy and filled with white sand. As you sink into deeper relaxation, allow the sand to flow out of every pore and tissue of your body.

For a few minutes succumb to deeper and deeper relaxation. Let go completely and visualize your body and mind floating away from you, merging with the infinite spirit. Finally, take a few deep breaths, and sit up slowly.

BENEFITS

You feel refreshed and relaxed.

Aches and pains are relieved.

Complete Relaxation combats both fatigue and insomnia.

It tones the entire body, including the facial muscles.

BREATHING EXERCISES

The mechanics of Yoga breathing are completely opposite to our everyday breathing, in which we suck in the stomach as we inhale and release it as we exhale. In Yoga breathing we push out the abdomen as we breathe in, lowering the diaphragm and thereby providing the lungs with the maximum space for expansion. With all this room to expand, the lungs can completely inflate, like balloons, down to the very bottom, something that rarely happens in routine breathing. An increased quantity of oxygen is carried to every inch of the lungs and throughout the system.

When you first begin to practice Yoga breathing, concentrate especially on this aspect of it, making sure you extend the abdomen as you inhale and contract it as you exhale. A good way to check yourself is by lightly resting your fingertips on your abdomen.

Another vital rule of Yoga breathing is to always inhale only through the nose, with the mouth closed. When we breathe through the mouth, we completely bypass the ingenious filtering system with which Mother Nature has equipped us. The combination of tiny hairs and mucous membranes in the nose strains out many of the impurities in the air, with the result that cleaner air is brought into the lungs.

Keep in mind that to breathe properly you must be able to control your breath at all times. Until now it has been rushing away from you in any old direction, but you must learn to master and direct it and to apply it at your will. Eventually, controlled breathing will become a natural habit. Until that time do not concern yourself with it as you practice the postures. Only breathe in and out through the nose with your mouth closed. Everything will come together naturally as you continue to practice the Breathing Exercises and the Postures.

Yoga Practice Breath

Yoga breath is divided into three parts: abdominal, intercostal or rib cage, and clavicular. We are going to isolate the three parts for practice.

Abdominal Breath

Place your hands lightly on your abdomen. Think of your abdomen as a balloon which you will fill with each inhale and totally empty with each exhale. Breathe in slowly through the nose. Feel the expansion of the abdomen and the air filling your lungs as one unified process. You will feel your fingers spreading apart from each other and your hands separating as your abdomen fills. Exhale slowly through the nose. Feel the air coming out and the contraction of the abdomen as one process. Eventually you will be able to totally empty yourself of wastes and toxins and consequently take in much more fresh air.

Repeat three times, each time trying to balloon out more with the inhale and push out more air with the exhale.

Intercostal Breath

Place your hands on the rib cage. Start by having your thumbs right up under the breasts, the heels of your hands on the sides of the rib cage and the fingers pointing toward the front. Now think of the rib cage as an accordion. Slowly inhale, expanding the ribs sideways. Feel the ribs separating from each other and the tissues spreading. Again think of the muscle expansion and the breath as one integrated movement. Then, slowly exhaling, let the ribs come together accordion-fashion. Strive to expel all air, wastes, and toxins.

Repeat three times.

Clavicular Breath

Gently place your fingertips on the clavicular area above the chest. Inhale slowly. From the inside, feel the back of the throat fill with air, while outside your hands feel for movement where they rest. Exhale slowly, emptying the lungs totally.

Complete Breath

You are now going to combine the three elements of abdominal, intercostal, and clavicular breaths, which you learned in Yoga Practice Breath, into one smoothly flowing "Complete Breath."

Sit in a comfortable cross-legged pose on the floor, holding your back, head, and neck in a straight line. Rest your hands loosely, palms up, on your knees. (In the beginning you may keep your fingertips lightly on your abdomen to make sure that you are performing the exercise correctly.) Empty your lungs before starting. To the count of eight, inhale deeply while pushing out your abdomen, rib cage, and chest, raising your shoulders slightly in a continuous flowing movement. Hold your breath in the back of your nose for eight slow counts. Lower your shoulders and start exhaling slowly to the count of eight, contracting your chest, rib cage, and abdomen. Some people find it more comfortable to exhale and contract first the abdomen, then the rib cage, and lastly the clavicular region. This is a matter of personal preference and is also correct. When you have completed exhalation, your abdomen and the surrounding area should be hollow. Pause ten seconds. Perform three times.

Try to gradually increase the length of inhalation and exhalation to ten seconds and the holding of the breath to the count of twenty. When you have comfortably reached this stage, slowly increase the period of holding your breath by five counts at a time. Remember, never strain to hold your breath longer than you can. The exhalation should always be controlled. The various steps of the exercise should be performed in a continuous flowing movement. Eventually learn to direct and hold your gaze at the tip of your nose.

BENEFITS

It purifies the blood, resulting in a healthy, glowing skin and a clear complexion.

It overcomes fatigue and restores vitality.

It improves mental alertness and clarity.

It acts as a tranquilizer for agitation, tension, and stress, and can also normalize breathing in palpitations.

The Complete Breath can be practiced either sitting, standing, or lying down at any time of the day in almost any situation. It can be used very appropriately to fill out any period of "dead" time, such as while you are waiting for a red light to change, sitting in the dentist's office, or standing in a line at a store. It can be done unobtrusively, without raising your shoulders in public. And it is enormously helpful to remember as an immediate tranquilizer in moments of acute anxiety or pain.

*Alternate Nostril Breathing or Pranayama
preceding Meditation*

This is also called sun and moon breathing. The right nostril takes in the sun breath and the left nostril the moon breath, representing the positive and negative currents respectively. Some teachers prescribe counting with this exercise, but I find counting distracting, and so advise my students to inhale and exhale as slowly as they possibly can without counting.

Sit in a comfortable cross-legged pose with your spine erect. Extend the thumb and last two fingers of your right hand, bending down the middle and index fingers. Even if you are left-handed, use your right hand. You will need practice to assume this hand position comfortably, but the result is more esthetic.

Close your right nostril with your right thumb. Inhale deeply through your left nostril. Immediately close your left nostril with your two extended fingers. Remove your thumb, but retain the breath for two seconds. Exhale as slowly as possible. Immediately inhale through your right nostril. Remove your fingers from your left nostril, retain the breath two seconds and exhale slowly. This is one round.

In practicing this exercise, always complete the round. Control the exhalation so that your breath doesn't rush away from you too quickly.

Start with three rounds. Gradually increase to six. As you become more adept at this exercise, begin retaining your breath with both nostrils closed, increasing the holding period to as long as is comfortable.

BENEFITS

By balancing the opposite currents in the body, Alternate Nostril Breathing helps restore equilibrium.

In the beginning, you will inhale and exhale more easily on

one side than the other because your nostrils are not balanced and the air is drawn up unevenly, but with practice you can achieve an even and controlled flow of air through each nostril, resulting in improved physical balance.

It promotes calmness and serenity by affecting the balance of the nervous system as well.

It relieves sinus conditions by helping to dissolve obstructions in the sinus cavity.

It facilitates unobstructed breathing by opening up the nasal passages. Regular practice will prevent nasal colds.

It relieves headaches.

It helps cure insomnia.

It prepares the body and mind for meditation, making them more receptive.

SPECIAL EXERCISES

As you become more and more involved in the Yoga process, firmer, stronger, more flexible, more supple, more in control of your breath and body, you may want to try out or add some of the postures from this section to your practice. Don't set goals which are unattainable. It is better to do fewer postures with total concentration and awareness than to attempt all the postures in the time that you allot to Yoga practice.

Choose the postures that appeal to you for a particular practice. As your body learns what the postures accomplish, it will help you make the choice according to its needs. It is very gratifying to see your inherent body wisdom grow as you practice Yoga.

As your body becomes really aware, on some days you will want to substitute some of the special postures for those in the Basic Practice Program.

On other days when you have more time, you may want to do the Basic Program, adding a special standing posture or

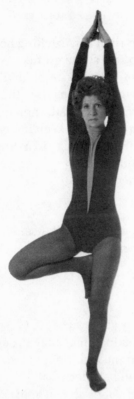

Stork

two to the standing section, a special sitting posture or two to the sitting section, etc.

Go ahead and explore these special postures, learn to enjoy them, and, most importantly, continue to advance as you practice.

Though the instructions include only one repetition, you may repeat each posture three times if you desire. If so, repeat on one side before going to the other side.

Stork

Balance firmly on the right leg, stretching and tightening all the muscles, and pressing the foot evenly into the floor as in the Dancer's Pose. Bending the left leg at the knee, slide the left foot up the inner right leg, catching hold of the ankle and bringing the heel to rest at the groin.

Press the left foot into the right thigh, and with equal pressure press the right thigh against the left foot.

When you are firmly balanced, inhale and raise the arms overhead. Breathing normally, keep intensifying the stretch. Hold for ten to thirty seconds. Exhaling, simultaneously lower the left leg and arms.

Repeat on the other side.

BENEFITS

Greatly enhances ability to balance.
Tones leg muscles, particularly inner thigh.
Slenderizes torso.

Arm Lock Stretch

Separate the legs by about two feet. Clasp the hands behind the back. Turn the left foot in about 45°, bending the left knee over the ankle. Turn the right foot out 90°. Keep the weight evenly distributed on both feet.

Turn the torso and pelvis so that your body is facing in the direction of the right foot. Lift the clasped arms as high toward shoulder level as you can, allowing the shoulder blades to come back and together.

Inhale slowly and expand the chest and rib cage as much as possible. Exhaling, stretch the lower back and slide the rib cage and torso forward and down, letting the head and neck dangle. Breathing normally, sink into the position, holding ten to thirty seconds. Make sure you keep weight evenly on both feet.

Inhaling, raise the torso and arms as one unit. When you are upright, exhale and lower the arms.

Turn and repeat on the other side.

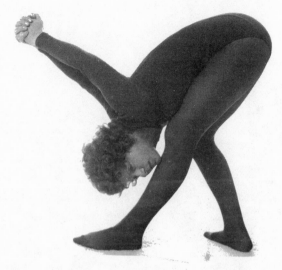

Arm Lock Stretch

BENEFITS

Tones and beautifies the chest.

Firms and strengthens the arms.

Tones the thighs.

Relieves aches and strains in the back and neck.

Reversed Triangle Pose

Separate the legs three to three and a half feet, arms at shoulder level. Turn the left foot in 60° and the right foot out 90°. Tighten and stretch the leg muscles, pressing the left heel and outer sole onto the floor (do not lose this leg stance as you continue).

Inhale. Exhaling, twist the torso to the right, placing the left hand outside the right foot or gripping the leg wherever possible. Straighten the right arm, gaze up at the right hand, and stretch the arms and shoulders intensely.

Breathing normally, hold ten to thirty seconds.

Inhaling, return to the starting position and repeat on the other side.

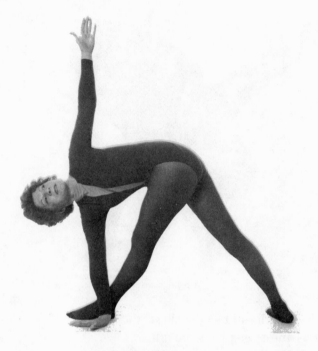

Reversed Triangle Pose

BENEFITS

Tones thigh and calf muscles and hamstrings.
Strengthens the spine and muscles of the back.
Invigorates abdominal organs.
Strengthens hip muscles.
Slenderizes and elasticizes waistline.

Ballet Pose

Come into a modified Stork, with the left foot at the level of
the right knee. Clasp the heel of the left foot (see picture).
Slowly straighten the leg sideways and stretch the right arm
to shoulder level. Keep the right and left leg muscles tightly

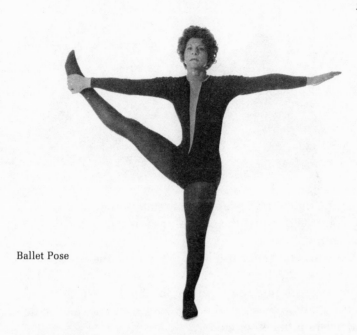

Ballet Pose

stretched, and let the weight evenly press the right foot onto the floor. Hold ten to thirty seconds. Exhaling, lower the leg and arms.

Repeat on the other side.

BENEFITS

Increases grace and ability to balance.

Tones the leg muscles, particularly those of the calf and inner thigh.

Extreme Alternate Leg Stretch

This is a variation of the Alternate Leg Stretch in which you bend the right knee and gently place the foot high up on the thigh. The knee of the bent leg should be comfortable and should touch the floor. Bring the right arm behind you and

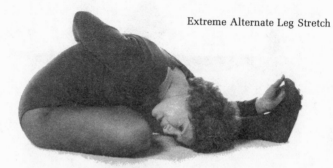

Extreme Alternate Leg Stretch

clasp the right foot. Tighten and stretch all the muscles in the left leg, straightening the back of the knee. Inhale. Stretch to the ceiling.

Exhaling, reach for the left foot, sliding the rib cage and torso forward. Make sure to keep the weight even on both buttocks. Sink into the position and hold ten to thirty seconds. Inhaling, come up slowly. Massage the knee and ankle.

Repeat on the other side.

BENEFITS

Same as the Alternate Leg Stretch, but more intense if your body is ready.

Sitting Twist

This is somewhat confusing to perform without an instructor. To help you keep track of where all your arms and legs belong, I've numbered the steps, but remember that what you're aiming for is a continuous flow of movement.

1. Sit erect with legs together and extended in front. Bend your right leg, bringing the foot up next to the left thigh.

2. Clasp your hands around your right ankle, lift your leg over the left thigh and place the foot parallel to the thigh.

3. Place your right hand directly behind you.

4. Lift your left arm over your right knee, and with your

Sitting Twist

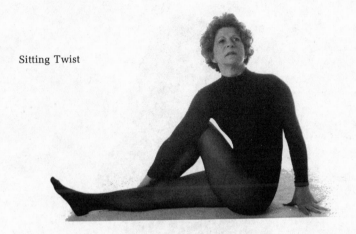

elbow pressing against your right thigh, firmly grip your left knee.

5. Exhale, twisting the upper part of your body to the right as far as you can, putting all the pressure on your right hand. Hold the pose for ten seconds, breathing normally.

6. Inhale as you untwist.

7. Untangle yourself and repeat on the left side.

BENEFITS

By locking the lower part of your body, you're free to twist the upper body to its utmost, enabling you to get rid of back pains, strains, kinks, and general discomfort.

Spinal flexibility is improved.

Twisting the body helps take inches from the waist.

You will experience immediate invigoration.

Posture Clasp

Fold the left leg and place it under the right thigh. Fold the right leg in at the knee, placing it on top of the left leg so that both knees are parallel.

Fold the left arm behind you at the elbow, moving the

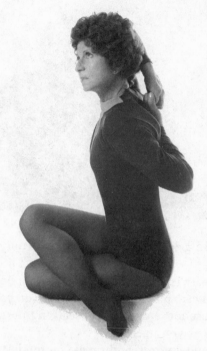

Posture Clasp

Hip Stand

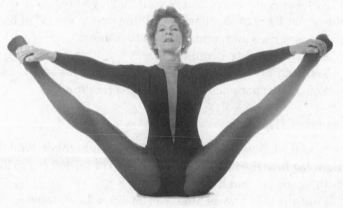

elbow as far up the back as possible. Fold the right arm over the shoulder with the elbow pointing up, behind the right ear. Try to clasp fingers, hands, or wrists. Use the clasp to press the spine toward the sternum and straighten the back. Breathing normally, stretch deeper into the pose. Hold ten to thirty seconds. Release the arms carefully.

Repeat on the other side. To practice for this position, hold a handkerchief or scarf with upper hand and reach for it with lower hand.

BENEFITS

Increases flexibility of knee, hip, elbow, wrist, and shoulder joints.

Improves posture.

Relieves tension in neck and upper back.

Hip Stand

Draw your knees up close to your chest. Bring your arms between your legs, and grasp the insides of your heels. Sit straight, inhale, and extend your left leg to the side, keeping your knees straight. Hold ten seconds, exhale, and relax. Do this three times with the left leg and three times with the right leg.

Now comes the tricky part. Hold on to both heels and lift both legs slightly. Straighten your back and establish balance in the region of your coccyx. Inhale. Now slowly lift both legs and extend them to the sides, keeping them as straight as possible, without rounding the back, as if you were doing a split off the ground. Hold for ten seconds, exhale, and relax.

Perform twice.

In the beginning you will surely roll backwards. Try not to laugh at yourself, but keep practicing until you achieve the proper balance.

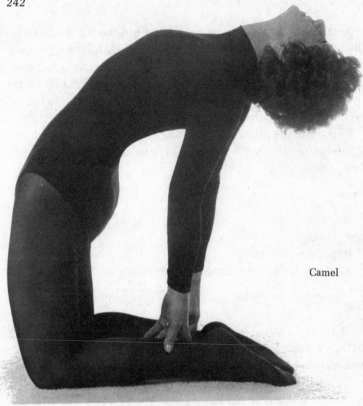

Camel

BENEFITS

This exercise is excellent for firming the thighs.

It relieves stiffness in the leg muscles, especially in the calves.

It strengthens the muscles in the upper back.

It promotes balance and coordination.

It tones the abdomen.

Camel

Kneel and sit on your heels. Hold your ankles or your heels, and raise your trunk, putting all your weight on your hands.

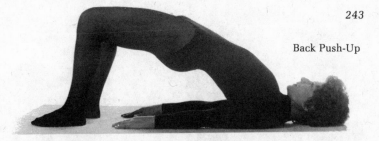

Arch your upper back. Tighten your buttock muscles and push your pelvis as far forward as possible. Let your head hang back. Hold, breathing normally, for ten to thirty seconds. Exhaling, sit down slowly.

If you find this position too uncomfortable, separate your legs about twelve inches and sit between them. Place your hands on the floor behind your feet, and push up.

BENEFITS

Flexibility of the back is increased.
Muscles of the bust and chest are firmed.
Front thigh muscles are toned, strengthened, and stretched.

Back Push-Up

Lie down, arms at your sides, palms down. Bend the knees and place the feet close to the buttocks. The feet should be parallel and about twelve inches apart.

Exhaling, raise your back one vertebra at a time, starting at the tailbone. Placing the weight on your shoulders, soften the back of the neck and gently press it onto the floor.

Expand the rib cage. Tighten the buttocks, and push the pelvis up.

Breathing normally, hold ten to thirty seconds.

Inhaling, come down one vertebra at a time. Press the small of the back into the floor for a count of eight before releasing the hips.

Repeat three times.

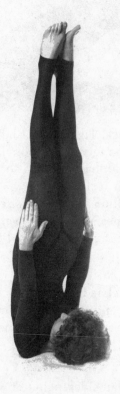

Extreme Shoulderstand

It is an excellent preparation for the Shoulderstand.
It aligns the spine and improves flexibility.
It strengthens the lower back.
It allows the organs to rest in the correct places.
It slenderizes the legs and torso.

Extreme Shoulderstand

When you have achieved the Shoulderstand with the arm clasp, you may unclasp the arms and raise the hands one at a time, placing the palms on the thighs.

Stay in the pose for one minute or longer, and return to the

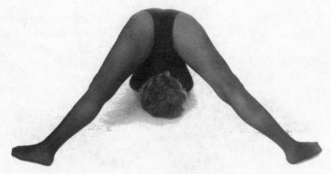

Split-Leg Plough Variation

supported Shoulderstand. Roll out or go into the Plough or a Plough variation.

BENEFITS

The entire body is toned by an increase in the flow of blood and by the elimination of toxin-forming waste matter.
Strengthens all back muscles.

Split-Leg Plough Variation

Proceed into the Plough with an arm clasp. Separate the legs as far as possible. Turn the toes out and press the soles to the floor.

Hold, breathing normally for one minute. Either roll out or go into another Plough variation.

BENEFITS

Same as Plough, with more toning to the thighs and intensified work on the lower back and neck.

Shoulder Twist/Knees to Shoulder Plough Variation

Proceed into the Plough, supporting the back with the hands or with an arm clasp. Walk the legs to one side of the

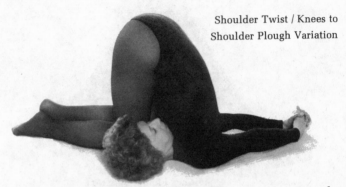

Shoulder Twist / Knees to
Shoulder Plough Variation

head. Slowly bend the knees, bringing them to rest against the shoulder.

Hold for one minute. Walk the legs back to the Plough and correct your posture and grip. Then repeat on the other side.

Return to the Plough. Either roll out or try the Complete Spine Stretch.

Complete Spine Stretch

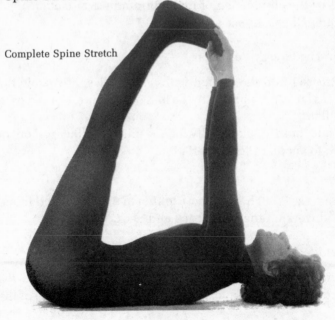

Pelvic Stretch

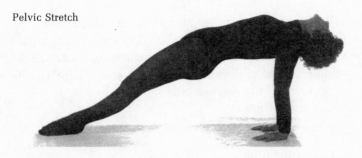

BENEFITS

Same as the Plough, with intensified work on back, waist, and thighs.

Complete Spine Stretch

Reaching your arms overhead, clasp your toes, keeping your legs straight. Start to roll out until the whole spine, even the tailbone, is on the floor. Press the lower spine onto the floor and tighten knees. Hold about thirty seconds.

Gently release your grip. Place your hands palms down on the floor. Keep the lower back glued to the floor and, exhaling, lower the legs. Relax.

BENEFITS

Increases spinal agility and flexibility.
Strengthens and relaxes the lower back.
Loosens calf muscles.

Pelvic Stretch

Sit up straight with your legs together in front of you. Place your hands flat on the floor about five inches behind you, with the fingers pointing sideways away from your body. With arms straight and heels pressing onto the floor, inhale, and slowly raise yourself off the floor. You should raise your pelvis as high as you can, your back should be arched, feet flat on the floor, and head back. Your weight should be supported by your hands and feet. Hold this position for five seconds, breathing normally. Come down slowly and exhale. Gradually increase hold to ten seconds.

Repeat three times.

BENEFITS

It firms hips, thighs, and buttocks.
It helps strengthen arms, shoulders, and back muscles.
It relieves tension in the neck and back.
It alleviates muscle cramps and spasms in the legs.

SUNRISE SALUTATION

The Sunrise Salutation, said to unite your body with the earth's elements and energy, is one of the best overall body conditioners. You stretch to the sun and the sky and melt into the earth in a flowing series of movements that exercise the entire body. You can build up to perform ten and eventually twenty complete Sunrise Salutations.

Proper breathing is essential because of extreme muscle exertion.

On days when you have very little time for practice, use the Sunrise Salutation and Total Relaxation in place of other practice.

You may wish to do a few Sunrise Salutations every morning—as the name implies—to start your day in harmony. It is a fantastic eye-opener, and you will find it wipes away those get-up blues and puts you into a high yet relaxed gear for your day. It induces superb flexibility for the entire spine and legs.

Sunrise Salutations done at a vigorous pace are an excellent

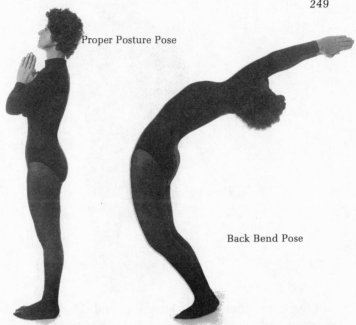

Proper Posture Pose

Back Bend Pose

cardiovascular toner and can be used as a form of aerobics. I encourage you to include some form of aerobics in your daily life (Sunrise Salutations, five to ten minutes of jumping rope, a good brisk walk at a steady pace, climbing up and down stairs in lieu of elevators, dancing, bicycling, jogging, etc.).

Following is a list of poses which, when put into a flowing sequence, will constitute a Sunrise Salutation. Please be careful to learn the Proper Posture Pose, as this is the only place I have described correct posture in great detail, and I urge you to concentrate on it and use it as a preparation for all standing poses.

Proper Posture Pose

Stand with your weight evenly distributed on the balls and heels of both feet, the inner soles pressed together, the ankles

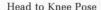
Head to Knee Pose

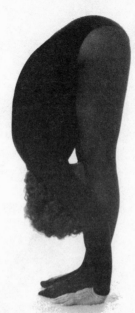

and the upper inner knees touching, and the muscles above the knees tightened and lifted. Press the upper thighs together and tuck the buttocks under.

The ankles should be parallel to the floor, and your weight should be aligned over the middle of the feet. The knees should be directly over the ankles. Stretch the entire legs upwards, especially the inner leg muscles. Relax the abdominal area; tighten the lower back and the buttocks.

The spine is straight, the rib cage is expanded, and the shoulders are completely relaxed. Place the arms at the sides of the body.

The above is proper Yoga posture. For purposes of the Sunrise Salutation, press both palms together under the chin as shown.

Back Bend Pose

Inhaling, stretch the arms up, arching the upper back from the waist and keeping the buttocks tight and tucked under.

One Leg Back Pose

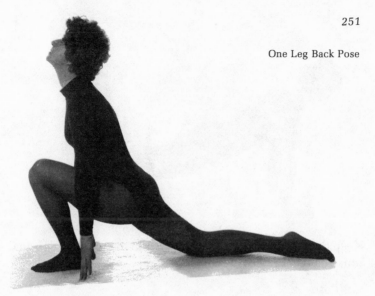

Head to Knee Pose

Exhaling, straighten and stretch your lower back and slide your torso down your legs. Place the hands on the floor on either side of the feet. There is little sense in doing the Sunrise Salutation until you have reached this state of flexibility. The hands remain in this position for the entire set of positions.

One Leg Back Pose

Inhaling, bend one knee as you slide the other leg back. Allow your body weight to stretch and strengthen the legs. At the same time, stretch the torso. (The leg you have moved back is the leg you will bend forward when you get to the second One Leg Back Pose of your Salutation.)

Wheelbarrow Pose

Holding your breath, place both palms on the floor, turn the toes under, and stretch the other leg back into a Wheelbarrow or push-up position. Do not allow the elbows to turn out.

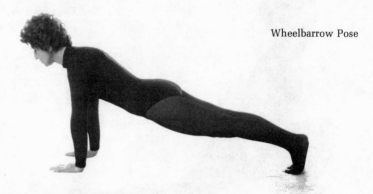

Wheelbarrow Pose

Keep the spine in a perfectly straight line and the abdominal muscles contracted.

Cat Pose

Exhaling, still keeping the elbows tucked in, and turning the toes back, bend the knees and lower the chest and chin to the floor, between the hands.

Cobra Pose

Inhaling, slide the body through the arms, keeping the chest on the floor, into a modified Cobra, with the elbows in.

Jackknife or Dog Pose

Exhaling, turn the toes under again and, using the arms, push the whole body as one unit onto the heels, pushing the head through the arms.

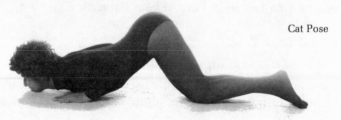

Cat Pose

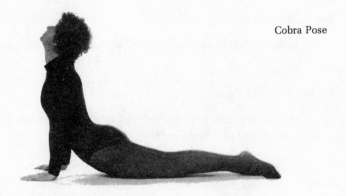

Cobra Pose

Now you are going to reverse the first four positions.

One Leg Back Pose

Inhaling, bend the knee and move the leg forward between the hands into the One Leg Pose.

Head to Knee Pose

Exhaling, simultaneously bring the other leg forward and slide the torso down the legs.

Jackknife or Dog Pose

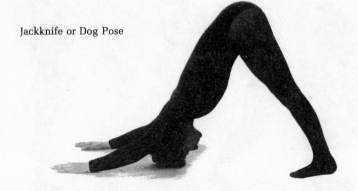

Back Bend Pose

Inhaling, stretch up and back, buttocks tight and tucked under.

Proper Posture Pose

Exhaling, return to Proper Posture Pose with the arms bent. Repeat on the alternate side.

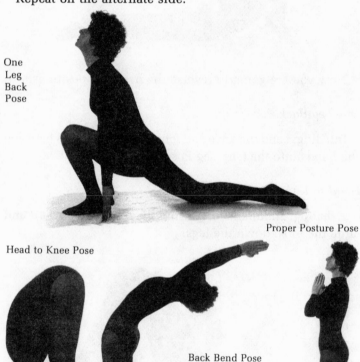

One
Leg
Back
Pose

Proper Posture Pose

Head to Knee Pose

Back Bend Pose

ADVANCED EXERCISES

(not to be attempted without instruction)

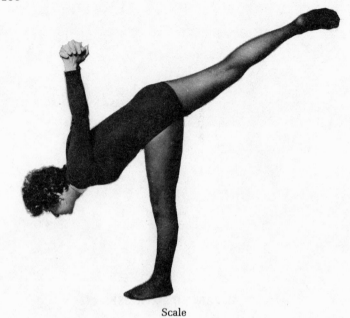

Scale

Lateral Angle Pose

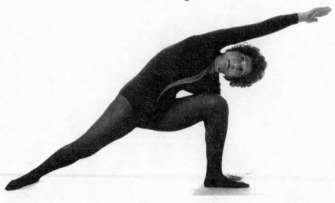

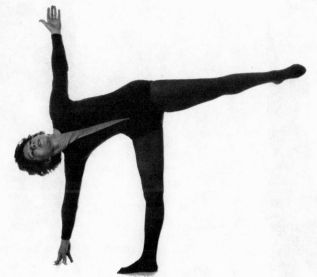

Extreme Ballet Pose

Reversed Lateral Angle Pose

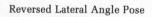

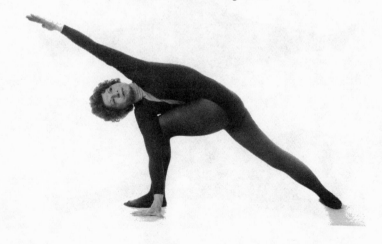

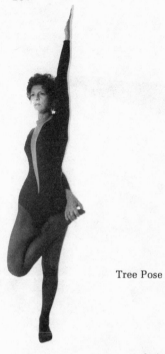

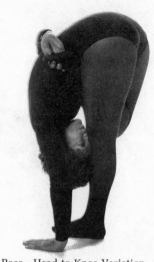

Tree Pose—Head to Knee Variation

Tree Pose

Split-Leg Forward Stretch

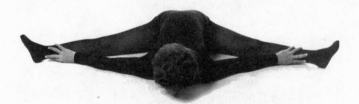

Split-Leg Side Stretch

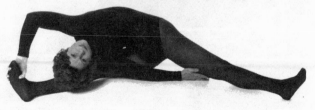

Toe Balance

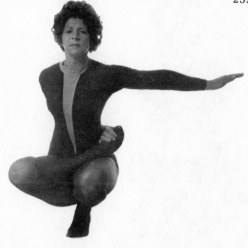

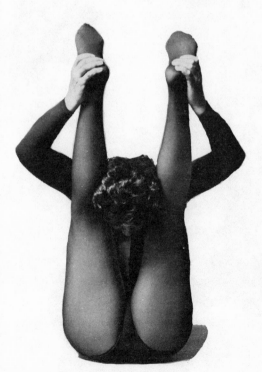

Extreme Hip Stand

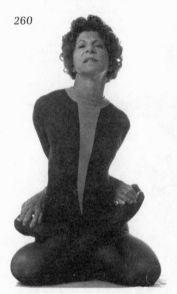

Bound Lotus Pose

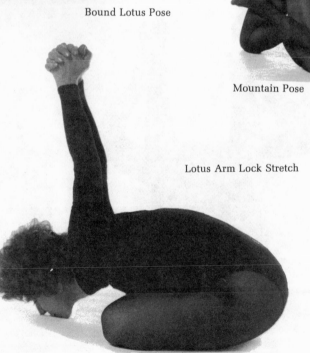

Mountain Pose

Lotus Arm Lock Stretch

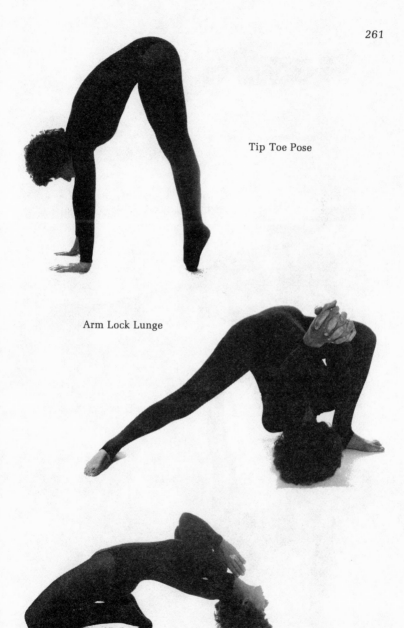

Tip Toe Pose

Arm Lock Lunge

Back Bend Toe Pose

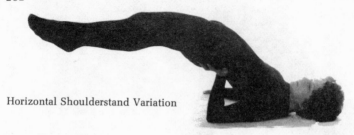

Horizontal Shoulderstand Variation

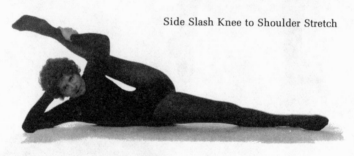

Side Slash Knee to Shoulder Stretch

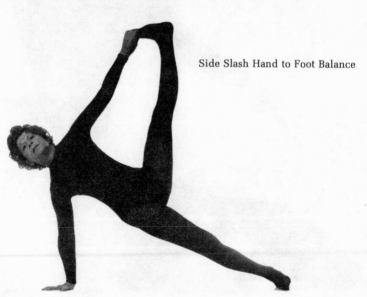

Side Slash Hand to Foot Balance

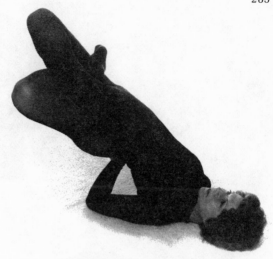

Horizontal Lotus Shoulderstand Variation

Graceful Pose Shoulderstand Variation

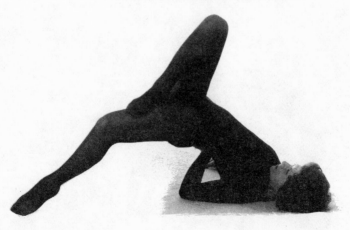

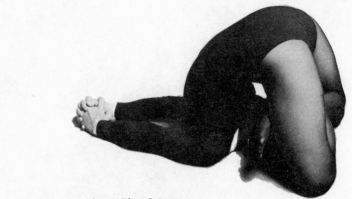

Lotus Plough Variation

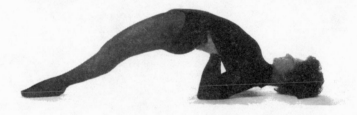

Bridge

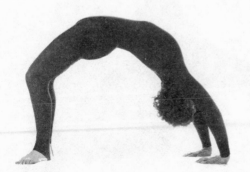

Wheel

Crow

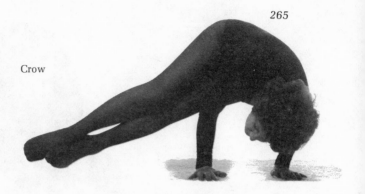

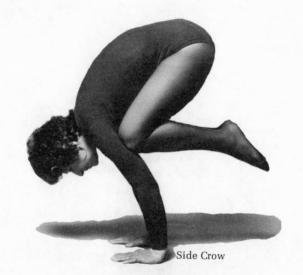

Side Crow

Peacock

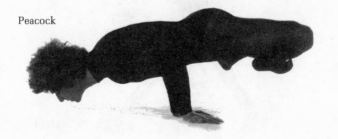

Tripod Variation

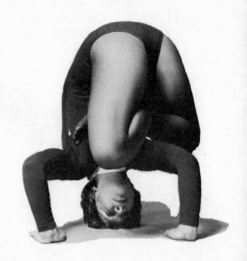

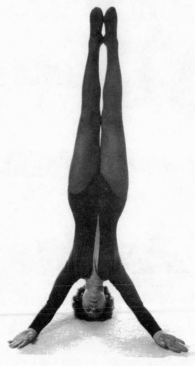

Wrist Headstand Variation

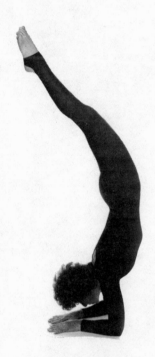

Scorpion (Forearm Pose)

INDEX